MW01110090

Dr. Sofia Costa is an author, artist and reiki master with a doctorate in physical therapy. In 2020, she self-published her first book, *The End of Back Pain: The Secret to Gaining Relief and Staying Active*.

Dr. Sofia was born in Puerto Rico to a family of artists, healers, shamans and medicine men and women, allowing her to gain access to ancient wisdom and spiritual practices that amplify Heart-Earth connection. She integrates the art of alchemical medicine through movement, breathwork, sound meditation, energy healing, and handcrafted creations.

Dr. Sofia's passion is guiding people on a heart-centred journey to alchemize fears, integrate a new way of being, and embody the power of who they are so they can strengthen their connection to Self, Earth, Lineage and Love.

To live wholeheartedly is Dr. Sofia's intention.

To my family, I love you. Thank you for believing in me and supporting my life's purpose.

To every person I've crossed paths with, thank you for being a catalyst for me to dive into the unknown within, so I can heal and understand who I am, rise in love, and experience a wholehearted life.

Dr. Sofia Costa

The Power of Being Known: A Heart-Centered Journey Connecting to Self, Earth, Lineage, and Love

AUSTIN MACAULEY PUBLISHERS™

LONDON • CAMBRIDGE • NEW YORK • SHARJAH

A CIP catalogue record for this title is available from the British Library.

ISBN 9781035811069 (Paperback)
ISBN 9781035811076 (Hardback)
ISBN 9781035811090 (ePub e-book)
ISBN 9781035811083 (Audiobook)

www.austinmacauley.com

First Published 2023
Austin Macauley Publishers Ltd®
1 Canada Square
Canary Wharf
London
E14 5AA

Table of Contents

.

The power of being known is an awareness of self,
and an understanding of who you are and why you're here.
The power exists in the space of stillness.
Be still, feel, ask, listen, breathe, receive, and know.
Connect to the beat of your heart.
Feel the present moment with the essence of your presence,
and accept life as is wholeheartedly.
Receive your self in this now moment.
Receive love from deep within for love is the power of being
known and love is a power worth knowing.
Be still, feel, ask, listen, breathe, receive,
and know.

Dr. Sofia Costa

A Letter from the Author

Dear Reader,

Thank you for being here in this now moment.

The unfolding of this book came to me in November 2021 while I was meditating between two trees at a family-owned homestead in Mt. Shasta, CA.

That morning I felt the book was ready to be birthed. I expressed this feeling with the host, a single mother I was renting the studio from, as she was milking a goat. She, too, felt the readiness of the birthing of the book and without hesitation said, "Go meditate between those two trees and don't leave until you receive everything you need to write this book." She stopped milking the goat, grabbed a blanket and we walked towards the trees where she laid the blanket down on the ground. I laid down, closed my eyes, and surrendered.

And immediately, I saw in my mind's eye the title of the book and the entire content of the book unfolded. The book's intention, the wisdom, and medicine – an all-encompassing experience – rushed in for me to receive. And moments later, I felt a breeze lightly touch my skin as if it were a sign that the meditative process was complete.

I opened my eyes, sat up, and saw all the goats staring at me with their alien-looking eyes.

Stood up and walked across the field towards the studio with a readiness to write. Ascended the stairs, opened the door, and entered the space where the book came to life.

Opened my laptop and the sacred words began to flow through me as if it was all meant to be.

This book was written with the intention of guiding you on an inward journey towards your heart – because heart-first connection is the medicine for feeling more present, supported, and loved. Heart-first connection carries wisdom that can be passed on as the legacy of love. Heart-first connection brings you home to know your Self and in knowing yourself, you get to return to love every single time.

Love heals.
Love connects.
Love unites.
Love is who you are.

In this book, I share the wisdom and medicine of my life's experiences that have brought me closer to my heart, plus stories from dear friends of mine that have experienced a catalyst for them to dive deeper into themselves so they can heal, feel more connected, and live wholeheartedly.

May this book support your heart-centred journey to connect to Self, Earth, Lineage, and Love.

I see you.
I hear you.
I feel you.
And I love you.

– Dr. Sofia Costa

Foreword

Dr. Chad's Journey

What was the catalyst in your life for you to know yourself on a deeper level and how has your life changed since you chose to dive in and explore within?

The decision for me to dive deeper into myself was in a way like a pot of water that simmers its way up into boiling over the top. There were feelings going on inside of me that had sparked up symptoms of unease, anxiety, confusion, insecurity, and even to a point of physical symptoms of disease for quite some time.

I would shake them off, distract myself, or just muster my way through it and still be able to accomplish the tasks at hand. They just kept on building and coming a little more up to the surface, causing painful situations to myself. I started to address them slowly once Sofia Costa made me aware of some of these things and allowed me some comfort to discuss and/or express these feelings.

Before then I felt shame, fear of judgement, the burden of bringing my issues onto others, or even overall ego to bury these things in. I slowly started investigating into what I was feeling, who I was, why these things were happening, why I would act in certain ways even though that was not my intention or holding me back from pursuing the things I wanted in life. I was even at times uncertain what I wanted or that I was broken in a way as things did not make sense. I would make small strides towards improvement or clarity and either ego, fear, or distracting myself with other things I would fall back into thinking I was okay.

I had been able to be extremely disciplined in multiple things in my life and figured I could just do the same with the emotional/psychological/spiritual aspects of my life. I figured I would just declare that I would stop doing the self-destructive behaviours, implement routine such as meditation, journaling, waking up early, getting out into nature more, eating healthier, and exercising more. I had made some progress in my career that had earlier given me stress, I had met and started dating someone that I really loved, I felt to be in really good physical health, and on the surface would seem pretty healthy.

Things then started to heat up, more challenging aspects of work began to increase, my family started to have some issues that I felt the need to take on, some insecurities that were deep in me that I wasn't fully understanding were brought to the surface in the relationship I was in, and I just kept on adding more on with excessive exercise, eating strategies, and feeling the need to learn and do more. Self-doubt was coming in hard, and I started to pull away from my relationship in ways as I was afraid, I wasn't good enough; I took on the problems of my patients and everyone around me; I started to get chest pains, shortness of breath, my libido was completely gone and even the ability to get aroused which brought on more shame.

I wasn't able to concentrate and the physical and mental abilities that I was proud of and were strengths of mine were deteriorating. I gained weight, had no drive, was just a shell of myself and instead of seeking help, talking with people about how I was feeling, and my fears I just went farther inward. I pushed it all down, I isolated myself, I didn't want to be a burden, and I just went harder into the discipline portion of trying to do certain tricks or things to get better.

The sad thing is that I was able to get rid of some of the physical symptoms and in my mind thought I had overcome things once again. But the doubt, isolation, pulling away, shame, insecurity, and fear was still there, and self-destructive behaviours started to peak their head in again.

After a small breakdown I decided to seek some help and work with a therapist, whom I really felt comfortable with. In my mind I thought I would do some work and it would fix the problem and I would be good to go. As with most things, dramatic changes happen at the beginning which allows you to feel good and think, damn I am good to go. That overconfident feeling of I can slow it all down and get right back into the game. This is when the water boiled over.

I was given another chance with my girlfriend and had an amazing experience with her and went home and out of the blue the self-destructive actions came out of nowhere, like something else was at the control of me. This led to emotionally hurting the girl I loved so much. That was the moment in which I decided enough was enough. It was one thing if I was the victim of my actions, decisions, and thoughts but for it to have a negative effect on someone I loved and cared for I would not allow that to happen. I was at my perceived rock bottom. I had ruined a relationship that I had cared so much about, hurting her in the process, I was drained of energy, I had no confidence, I was not enjoying life the way

I used to, I was completely lost, and physically I felt like shit. That day in which is engrained in my brain for many reasons was the day I made the decision to go all in and work through all of the inner turmoil that was allowing me to ruin my life. I would dive deep into therapy; I would look into other methods that would allow me to better understand who I was and what was going on. I was open to any uncomfortable feelings that may arise. This decision, in my opinion, may have been the best one I have ever made.

Since that decision, things have improved in my life in such a dramatic way. It was like anything in life that is worth it and delivers great results, very difficult. There were many ups and downs, times in which I felt like throwing in the towel, times in which I felt completely unstable and like life was chaotic. But as I sit here writing this I feel more like a human being and comfortable with myself than I have ever felt. It has greatly improved the relationships in my life, including the one I have with myself. It has allowed me to have more energy to pursue the things I enjoy and the ability to actually see what I enjoy and not just doing to fit in. It has allowed me to be more aware of emotions that I am feeling and take the time to understand why I am feeling them. Hell, it has allowed me to feel and not be numb to everything as I was so used to pushing things down and not expressing them. It has given me the ability and confidence in myself to build my career and business the way I want to and handle the constant stress and pressure that being an entrepreneur brings. It has allowed me to become a better physician as I see the effects that emotional/spiritual/psychological turmoil can bring and makes me more aware of how all systems play off of each other and to look at all aspects of the human in front of me. It has allowed me to handle the stresses the world brings in a more compassionate light and be more patient with myself and others.

I still have the drive to operate at a high level and put a lot on myself, but I am much more forgiving and allow myself to take time and just relax and enjoy life, which in turn allows me to operate at an even higher level. I am able to learn and understand things even quicker than before and my overall physical health may be the best it has ever been with doing less. I feel like I truly understand who I am, what I value in life, and am accepting of myself and my past mistakes which brings with it a confidence in which I have never experienced. I actually have the self-worth to take care of myself and my needs, which as corny as it sounds, has allowed me to better be able to help others. I am excited to see where the remainder of this journey takes me and the more I can learn about myself. Extremely grateful for this opportunity, as I am not sure where I would be today if I did not make the decision to dive in and stick with it.

Part I
Knowing Your Self Begins by Knowing Your Cells

Introduction

The power of being known begins with knowing your Self- knowing *all* aspects of your Self – on a deep cellular level.

Why on a deep cellular level?

Because your cells hold DNA and DNA holds information – about your past, present, and future; about your ancestors, where you came from, and information about who you are and what you're made of.

You are a cell.

One cell of many.

Together, co-creates your entire being.

The co-creation of your entire being began with one cell.

One cell carrying all the wisdom, medicine, intelligence that you need to breathe, live, and experience this life.

And you have the power to choose how you'd like to experience living this life that's been specifically designed for you – uniquely created for you to heal and awaken to the truth of who you are and your destiny.

And it begins by knowing you are one cell – one cell of many – and the co-creation of your entire being began with one cell. And it's time to know your Self – all aspects of your Self – because there's power in being known, and it begins by journeying inward.

'The power of being known' was first spoken to me during a conversation with a dear friend of mine who I refer to as my California Mother. On November 4, 2021, I called her crying because I received news earlier that morning that a close friend of mine of 13 years died from a car accident. I told my California Mother that I heard my friend's voice tell me 'keep going' as I was crying on the floor wondering what to do next. At the time, I was road tripping solo along California which began in San Diego with the intention of ascending towards Mt. Shasta before traveling to Texas to visit my family. –

So, on the floor, tears flowing through me, I asked myself, "Do I stop my California journey and return to Texas now to be with my family? What do I do?"

Then there was a pause of silence and I heard my friend's voice tell me, "Keep going."

When I shared this experience with California Mother, she expanded on what the voice said to me, "Keep going with what's inside of you. There is power in being known. And that sounds like the title of your next book."

Her words resonated. Every single cell in my body vibrated.

Keep going with what's inside of you. There is power in being known.

And that's been the theme of my journey – continuing to acknowledge what's going on inside of me because there's power in being known – deeply knowing myself as priority and allowing others to know me.

To be honest, it's easy to hide when experiencing grief and heartache. It's easy to put up walls to guard myself from feeling. It's easy to hold it all in and hide my vulnerability.

It's easy because that's something I was good at for many years. But how is that truly living? How is that allowing myself to know *me* – all of me – and honour the design and creation of my being?

Hiding in grief, heartache, guilt, shame and fear didn't allow me too truly live. I could hardly breathe and felt pain in my body.

But it took grief, heartache, guilt, shame, and fear to crack me wide open – because it triggered me to feel all of the emotions and learn from it, then allow the emotions to move through me with awareness, acceptance, courage, grace, and peace. Those lower vibrational emotions (grief, heartache, guilt, shame, and fear) no longer had power over me – and that moment of empowerment happened when I chose all of me, when I chose to dive deeper, and get to know *all* aspects of me – of who I AM – and what's my destiny.

I dove into the unknown deep inside of me and dove in daily because surrendering and trusting opens the portal, the gateway into the Self, the all-encompassing Self.

Surrendering leads to resurrection.

The unknown is within you. You no longer need to fear it nor escape from it. You're safe.

Time to make the unknown, known, and connect to the power of being known.

Chapter 1
You Are One Cell One of Many

Every cell in your body connects and communicate with each other, and together, they transfer information via electricity and energy.

Each cell has its own programming with specific functions for you to move your body, eat and digest your food, breathe, think, feel, create, sleep, recall memories, play music, sing, and connect with all of Mother Earth's creatures and creations.

Every cell is designed with purpose on purpose which means *you* are designed with purpose on purpose. There are no mistakes when it comes to the design of *you*, to the design of your cell(s), to the design of your body, to the design of your life.

The cell produces its own energy source, holds genetic information and expression, contains generational beliefs, wisdom, trauma, and medicine, and it's all influenced by your thoughts, emotions, words, and lifestyle choices. The cell remembers everything. And can shift, change, transform, die, and regenerate – a continuous cycle occurring deep within you.

The cell absorbs everything and uses it as fuel to perform and do its job, to fulfil its purpose of keeping you alive. The cell has the ability to send signals when you feel pain, stress, heartache, and support you with needing to run from a dangerous situation, heal wounds, repair the gut lining every 2–3 days, circulate hormones, repair tissue damage, etc. The cell has a powerful role in the creation of your of being and has its own intelligence to support you with what you need to stay alive and experience life in totality.

And you get to choose how you'd like to experience your life. You get to program your cells to fulfil your life's purpose and experience your heart's desires. The cells function and fulfil their purpose best when you intend to heal, be present, connect to your heart and body, love your Self with thoughts, words, and intentional actions that nourish your soul, free yourself from ancestral trauma, dedicate each day to feeling every emotion and living authentically in full expression, dive deeper into knowing your cell (Self) so you can fulfil your purpose with gratitude, compassion, courage, strength, and freedom.

The journey begins by connecting to the cells, the cells programmed with an intelligence to support you with everything you need.

Fuel your cells with love.
Love is a frequency that heals and unites.
Love is a vibration that sparks light.
Love is medicine that repairs your body and soul.
Love is what designed every cell to create you.
Love is the essence, the true essence of all of you.
Love is the energy that's eternal and never runs out.
Love flows, like water, infinite and ever-evolving.
Love is who you are.

And it's time to wake up and remember.

Every cell holds wisdom and medicine that are waiting to be unlocked and awakened. And connecting to the heart is the key to gaining access to the truth, love, and healing we tend to search for outside of ourselves. The heart is the first organ to be created while you're in your mother's womb and chosen to be first for a divine reason.

This book is a journey of my personal story of how I transitioned from self-abandonment to self-empowerment, from self-doubt to self-love, from heartache to heart freedom, from fearing love to embodying love, from gripping onto what felt comfortable to letting go, and surrendering, trusting I have everything I need within me because I AM love and love is the true essence of who we are.

As you continue to read on, you'll discover passages from my journal written in italics, introspective practices that can support you with feeling present within your heart and body, invitations to connect deeper into your Self and Mother Earth, plus inspirational stories from people I crossed paths with.

The book guides you on an inner exploration, emphasizing on the heart as your internal compass so you can return to love and arrive home.

Chapter 2
You Receive What You Believe

Every emotion, every moment, every breath serves a purpose. And I understand that's challenging to believe because it can feel painful to experience the darker side of life.

But it took darkness for me to find the light – the light deep inside.

Darkness is needed for us to shine light on.

Darkness serves a purpose for us to open our eyes and wake up.

Wake up to the lessons. Wake up to the gifts and blessings. Wake up to the wisdom. Wake up to the medicine.

Every emotion, every moment, every breath serves a purpose.

Every experience is a catalyst whether to hide or expand, whether to dim our light or shine brighter, whether to react in anger or pause and listen – everything is a catalyst, and we get to choose how we want to embrace it and experience it.

The catalyst that shifted my life

Summer of 2017 was a catalyst for me – so much so it felt like an oceanic wave of turbulence, one after the other, after the other – wiping out, unable to take back control and I lost myself – a part of me left me.

The big oceanic wave that was a catalyst for me was when I received news that my cousin died from a bus accident two days after celebrating his 43rd birthday.

My cousin was known for being a wild, free spirit – he allowed the wind of life carry him wherever he was needed. He created, painted, and danced to music. His presence and energy lit up every room he walked in. And I admired that about him. We were close growing up and shared stories relating to how different we felt within our family dynamic. He was the middle sibling of two brothers and I'm the middle sibling of two sisters. My cousin and I were the 'weird' ones because deep down we both knew we were destined for something more in this life, more than just working a 9–5 job, more than just waking up to hustle and pay bills, more to life than just feeling confined to societal programming.

My cousin travelled around the world, and he allowed his presence to be known.

His laugh, his light, his love. And he spread all his magic like glitter.

So, when he transitioned into the Heavens, I felt a part of me went with him.

And I forgot my why.

I forgot why I'm here.

I forgot who I AM.

At the time, I was working with clients in person, as a Doctor of Physical Therapy. And when I received the phone call of his passing, I was getting ready to teach a workshop on diaphragmatic breathing.

Which reminds me, that's what *I* needed. I needed to breathe. Breathe and remember to live my life and share my story.

But I couldn't share my story for some time because I felt paralyzed in heartache and grief and had yet created space to know about *my* story. I had to get to know my own story, connect to it, and experience the unfolding for me to share the wisdom and medicine with you now.

And that's challenging to do when you feel like you've lost a part of you.

During this time, I was also in a relationship – a brand new one.

We met 10 days prior to my cousin's passing at a workshop learning about energy frequency therapy. Looking back, learning about energy frequency therapy was the beginning of my journey of evolving beyond physical therapy.

And at first, the connection within the relationship seemed fine. We travelled well together, we shared similar interests, and enjoyed learning all things relating to the body, and our connection seemed to be going well during the first six months. Yet, I could strongly feel in my gut, something wasn't entirely right – something felt off inside of me and between us. And to be honest, I'll spare you the details. But I will add that the relationship experience felt turbulent like the ocean during a storm, and it seemed there were more storms than stillness.

The outer turbulence was a direct reflection of my inner turbulence of fears and emotions.

And I honestly believed this was as good as it was going to get for me. I thought I could make the relationship work. I thought I could save us and keep our relationship going. But deep down I was drowning, suffering in silence, struggling to keep it all together while I was navigating through the heartache and grief of my cousin's transition into the Heavens. And since I didn't allow myself to express my needs fully because I was afraid of being judged and abandoned, my inner world reflected into my outer world and most times, it wasn't pretty.

At the end of January 2019, after a year of living together, I approached him and said, "I'm not liking the person I'm turning into. I need to heal from everything that's been going on and I need to heal without you here. I choose me this time."

He respected my decision and a couple of days later, he got on a plane and left. And a new chapter began.

I began my eight-week journey of working with a colleague of mine, who was a certified relationship coach and RIM (Regenerating Images in Memory) therapist, because I no longer wanted to experience unhealthy relationships with myself, others, and even with money, and understood that if I desired healthier connections, I must explore within, acknowledge the fears, limiting beliefs, and emotions, heal my heart, and love every cell in my body.

During one of our phone sessions, fear of abandonment and a limiting belief that I wasn't deserving of love came up to the surface. We discovered that the fear and limiting belief originated from when I felt unloved and abandoned throughout my childhood because my parents were very busy working as medical physicians and were highly stressed most of the time. As a young child, I perceived myself as unloved and abandoned every time my parents left the house to go to work. And I subconsciously created a belief, *I'm not deserving of love.* The energy of that limiting belief vibrated at a low frequency deep inside of me, altering my perception of how I viewed myself and others. And since, I was seeing life through the lens of unworthiness.

To shift my perception from abandonment to love, and recreate a new belief, I was guided by my relationship coach/therapist to connect with my inner child. Space was held for my younger Self to feel safe, loved, and supported to express her feelings of heartache. I expressed her words out loud with tears in my eyes. I visualized myself embracing her in my arms and reminded her that she is loved and deserving of love. I expressed to my younger Self that it wasn't Mom and Dad's fault for working so much because they had their own beliefs and reasons why. My parents being busy didn't mean I wasn't loved. And by the end of the session, younger Sofia found love, the love she had been searching for, deep inside her heart. And from the space of love, she forgave herself and parents.

I witnessed another facet of darkness today. And I'm learning to forgive myself and love myself through this phase.

It's a hard lesson. A challenging journey – facing the darkness within myself and choosing to forgive and love myself anyway.

The darkness won't last forever because the light switch just needs to be turned on.

The fear won't last forever because love overrides it all and brings healing to those parts of me that's been needing it.

I no longer need to fill a void nor run away.

I'm worth loving and being loved. I'm worth being forgiven and tended to with a nurturing heart.

The cosmic skies and the Full Moon are pulling things out of me, bringing a lot to the surface to be faced, felt, forgiven, and loved.

All I can do is surrender.

And breathe through it – while staying connected to the present – loving every single cell of my body.

The catalyst that changed my life inspired a heart-centred journey of diving deeper into my Self, to explore what's been hidden in the darkness. From self-abandonment to self-love, a journey of connecting to my heart and listening to her whispers so I can heal from fears, emotions, and beliefs that were confining me from experiencing the richness of life wholeheartedly. A journey of no longer running away from myself and escaping from the discomfort of the past. A journey of surrendering and waking up to the truth. A journey of alchemy – learning, growing, healing, and returning to love – over and over again – continuously, because I'm worth knowing my own story of who I AM and why I'm here.

Invitation

What was a catalyst in your life that inspired you to heal, change, and evolve so you can love yourself again and live a more connected life? Reflect upon moments, travel back through time, and acknowledge that they happened for you. And celebrate yourself for gaining the courage, strength, and resilience to move forward and continue living this life. Celebrate your journey now.

Part II
Heart Connection
Connects You to All

Chapter 3
Tend to Your Heart,
She's Welcoming You Home

I cheated on my heart before my ex-boyfriend did in 2018.

I cheated on my heart when I didn't speak my truth, when I wasn't honest with myself, when I avoided listening to my heart's whispers, when I neglected to feel my emotions, when I stopped trusting my intuition, when I placed other people's needs before my own, and when I lost myself in the process.

I cheated on my heart before anyone else did.

And it wasn't my fault. I forgive myself for not knowing how to self-regulate emotions and connect to my heart.

It wasn't anyone's fault. I forgive them for not knowing how to self-regulate emotions and connect to their own heart.

As mentioned before, every moment, and every experience is a catalyst to dive deeper within because the outer world is a reflection of the inner world and vice versa.

So, yes, I'm grateful for the wave of catalysts, for the tears and heartache.

Each wave led me to *me* – deep inside of me.

Heartache shines light on moments when you didn't receive yourself fully. Moments when you self-abandoned to

33

escape and not feel, distracting yourself to numb out the pain, which fragmented pieces of your soul and you're left wondering why you feel tired with a void deep inside of you. A void needing to be filled with light and compassion, yet it's filled with fear, darkness, self-sabotaging thoughts, words, and actions. And you live out the belief that you're unworthy, not good enough, and underserving.

Heartache shines light on moments when you didn't receive yourself fully.

And now you get to create space of stillness and allow fragmented pieces of your soul to return – return home in your heart and body because you chose to stop escaping and connect to the parts of you you've been avoiding facing.

So, receive yourself in this now moment. Retrieve the parts of you that left because you didn't feel safe or supported. Allow the space of stillness to open your heart and feel the love, higher vibrational love, and receive.

Receive yourself fully. Receive this higher vibrational love and believe you are deserving to receive.

> *Receive your Self.*
> *Receive love.*
> *Receive healing.*
> *Receive.*
> *Breathe.*
> *And receive in this space of stillness.*

And the more I dove deeper inward, the more I got to know myself and realise my heart is worth being tended to.

I no longer wanted to cheat on my own heart.

I no longer wanted to abandon and neglect her.

34

For continuing to do so, creates more pain, stress, and a sense of unfulfillment.

I had to learn how to pour love into myself so that I can fulfil my divine purpose.

And to fulfil my divine purpose, I had to fill myself up with trust, compassion, forgiveness, and surrender. I had to dive into the unknown, the void within myself, and fill it up with my own love for self.

And in doing so, my heart is loved, seen, and heard. My heart gets to heal. And I feel more whole – all the bits and pieces that got lost along the way, I get to reclaim and love on every single aspect of *it* – the *it* that allows me to remember who I AM.

It took waves of catalysts to get to where I AM today. To be the woman I'm designed to be and choose that woman every single day.

Choosing me, receives you.

Choosing to know myself allows me to know *you*, see *you*, feel *you*, hear *you*.

For knowing myself, I get to know you. And you choosing to know yourself, you get to know me.

For we are ONE – all connected and free.

And it begins by tending to your heart and listening to her needs.

You can start now.

No need to wait.

Start now by placing one hand over your heart.

Feel her rhythm. Hear her beat.

Listen to her whispers.

And allow her to speak.

She's been waiting for you.

And right now, you can choose to connect to Her.

Open the door to your heart.

Walk in and feel her rhythm. Hear her beat.

Allow her warmth to embrace you.

She's welcoming you in.

Forgive yourself for ignoring her.

Forgive yourself in this now moment.

Allow her warmth to embrace you.

She's welcoming you in.

This is your home.

Here is where you belong.

This sacred space is what you've been searching for.

And now the door is open for you to step forward.

Walk in. Enter your home.

You're safe.

Breathe into this space – expand it even more.

Breathe out and receive your heart's divine love.

Feel her rhythm. Hear her beat.

Listen to her whispers.

And allow her to speak.

The answers are within you.

The truth is deep inside of you.

Release and let go.

And dive into the unknown and begin to know your self.

Journey inward. Tend to your heart.

She's welcoming you home.

You're safe.

Release and let go.

Feel her rhythm. Hear her beat.

You are now home.

Feel into this daily.

Experience your self by tending to your heart.

Deepen your connection and dismantle the walls.

There's nothing to fear.

There's nothing to worry about.

Your heart is here – always has and always will be.
Your heart was the first organ to be created. The first organ before the brain.

The heart beats because of an electrical spark. So, whenever you self-doubt, remember the power of your heart. And her power strengthens the more you connect to her. Designed with purpose on purpose, your heart is all knowing. She is the wisdom keeper of who you are and the medicine cabinet of your soul. She carries wisdom, intelligence, answers, solutions, comfort, love, compassion. She is your internal compass. And connects to the rest of your body.

Her energy circulates blood, messages, thoughts, feelings, and emotions. She carries memories and remembers everything. She pumps blood for you to breathe and live this life – a life you get to experience fully.

"The heart is the most powerful source of electromagnetic energy in the human body, producing the largest rhythmic electromagnetic field of any of the body's organs. The heart's electrical field is about 60 times greater in amplitude than the electrical activity generated by the brain. The magnetic field produced by the heart is more than 100 times greater in strength than the field generated by the brain and can be detected up to 3 feet away from the body, in all directions. …we have performed several studies that show the magnetic signals generated by the heart have the capacity to affect individuals around us." – HeartMath Institute, Science of the

Heart: Exploring the Role of the Heart in Human Performance.

The HeartMath Institute Research Centre has proven through 30 plus years of clinical research that the heart influences our awareness, intelligence, health, emotions, intuition, and perceptions. Connecting to your heart daily by placing your hands over your heart for a minimum of three minutes creates energetic and physiologic changes. And the electromagnetic field powers up like a fully charged cell phone to support the emotional and physical body, and Earth's magnetic fields. Common results from the research studies focusing on heart connection include feeling lighter, calmer, more present and connected, restful sleep, reduced levels of anxiety and depression, and better energy.

The heart's electromagnetic field creates a rippling effect. What you think, feel, and say travels beyond you – a power influenced by love or fear.

So, why not pause and connect to your heart daily?
Your heart invites you to.

Carine's Journey

What was the catalyst in your life for you to know yourself on a deeper level and love every single cell of your body?

I have mentors and spiritual teachers that have helped me and guide me to understand what love means. And the biggest catalyst for me wanting to love myself more is that I wanted to be in less pain. I realised that if I could be the energy that I wanted to receive, then I would be in less pain. So, In other words, if I wanted to receive more love or be more accepted and feel like I was part of a community, then I had to BE that – so I had to find a way to love others and give to others and be generous to others in order to feel loved.

And understand that I could love others the way that I want to be loved and in doing that, I learned what love was for me and feeling love from others.

So, the idea of self-love for me really is to understand that love is to give and to be generous and to be forgiving and to put it out there first and that includes myself – loving myself by loving others then creates this infinite loop of love where I feel I can give and receive.

My biggest catalyst is really to just get myself out of pain and not feel so limited and feeling small because I feel that when you don't feel love, you feel the contraction, you feel more fear, you feel more anxiety, you feel unable to do certain things; where if you're in this experience of feeling love, then it feels more infinite, there's more possibilities, there's more grace, there's more compassion, there's more forgiveness – there's more of life! And I wanted to be in that state more than the fearful, contracted state which doesn't give me the freedom that I've always to have in my life.

Being in pain, desiring freedom, and wanting to be a good person in the world has led me to want to love more and understand how I can utilise love in a healing way to benefit others and at the same time uplevel my life.

Your Body Isn't Broken.
The Connection to Your Body Is.

I've been fascinated by the heart ever since I was young, and the fascination began in 1999 when I was 16.

Two months after experiencing surgery on my left lower leg, I experienced migraines and heart palpitations. My father, a paediatrician then, scheduled an appointment for me to see a cardiologist for an examination to figure out why. The cardiologist discovered I was experiencing heart arrhythmias and recommended my heart to be monitored for seven days by wearing a holter (a heart rhythm recording device). I learned about electrocardiogram (ECG/EKG), how to put on the electrical leads on my body, and wore it all day every day, even during sleep, it was always with me. Seeing the leads and wires coming out of my body had me perceive myself as different and broken. I didn't understand what was going on with my body. I didn't know what my heart was trying to tell me.

After seven days, I returned to the cardiologist and I felt liberated, no longer needing to wear the machine. I no longer felt foreign or bionic. And now it was time for me to understand why my body experienced a lot of pain and discomfort. The EKG results from the holter revealed heart arrhythmia, which is an irregular heartbeat. The cardiologist expressed that it was normal for my age, and I'll eventually outgrow it.

Two months later, my back began to ache along the left side. I had trouble sitting, sleeping, walking, and received physical therapy for two weeks only to gain temporary relief. (To learn more on how I ended 15 years of back pain and supported many others, check out my first book called *The End of Back Pain: The Secret to Gaining Relief and Staying Active*).

So, here I am, at the age of 16, recovering from left leg surgery, an irregular heartbeat, and left sided back pain, desiring to play tennis and be active again, and at the same time, I deeply desired to be held, loved, seen, and heard so that I didn't feel alone navigating why my body felt broken. Journaling provided emotional support and I've been journaling ever since because magic happens when pen touches paper.

Lead with love.

My left leg reminded me to lead with love, and the scar and pain I felt and experienced along my left side was to teach me about love – self-love – to love every single cell of my body because I am worthy of my own love – to love within and lead with love.

All the heartache, grief, betrayal, and abandonment felt along the left side of my body was all wisdom for me, and medicine, to heal my heart.

Love heals all and all heal with love.

There is wisdom in everything – every second, every moment, every thought, every feeling, every emotion, every experience, every person you cross paths with – all hold wisdom for healing, for growth, for transformation.

The animals I've been seeing lately have been reminding me of that: butterflies, caterpillar, ladybug, and even the wind blowing through me, all relate to the healing, growth, and transformation I've been experiencing within because I chose to – I chose to embark on a self-healing journey.

At the age of 16, did I perceive that I didn't receive love when my body was hurting? Yes.

Did I perceive I was abandoned, left on my own to navigate the experience solo? Yes.

Did I perceive my body as ugly and broken? Yes.

And I received what I perceived.

And at the same time, did I believe I was going to get stronger? Yes.

And I received what I believed.

It was up to me to shift my beliefs and perception to experience a better reality – a more loving and supportive one – so I can feel more connected and liberate myself from the heartache of coping with a body I didn't understand yet.

The pain that I experienced at a young age was a catalyst for me to dive deeper into learning more about my body and how I can support others on their journey so they, too, can feel lighter, free, and connected in all ways – mind, body, heart, and spirit.

I attended Texas A&M University in College Station, TX to study Exercise Physiology. During my last year of my studies there, I learned all about the heart and cardiac rehabilitation which included the anatomy and physiology of the heart, how to read EKG reports, learn various heart conditions, and how to support one's recovery after heart surgery. Anything and everything about the heart, I got to learn – which was challenging and rewarding.

My last semester prior to graduating with my bachelor's, I interned for 12 weeks (6 weeks inpatient cardiac rehab, 6 weeks outpatient cardiac rehab). I got to help patients regain their strength and feel like they were alive again. I even got to observe a five-bypass cardiac surgery (among several other types of surgeries) and my fascination with the heart grew even stronger.

A common complaint I noticed among the patients in cardiac rehab was high levels of stress from overworking. Their lifestyle was go-go-go and they were unaware how to nourish themselves from the inside-out. They didn't sleep well and prioritised getting things done on their to-do list over slowing down and meditating (being present). They burned out and their heart gave out.

I also noticed they had low self-esteem by the way they carried themselves with a slouched posture and by their choice of words when describing their way of life. They didn't love their body. They didn't love the Self wholeheartedly and were malnourished.

Malnourished energetically, physically, mentally, spiritually, and emotionally because their bodies were carrying the heaviness of fears, limiting beliefs, heartache, shame, anger, guilt, and unworthiness; they were unconsciously living, asleep to the truth of who they are– a dissonance with Self, Earth, love, spirit, and their lineage.

Listening to the patients' stories, I couldn't help but realise that their symptoms related more to an emotional heartache rather than a physical one. And to be clear, I'm not dismissing the physiological aspect of heart defects and diseases. My intention is to add a perspective needed for deeper healing, a perspective that goes beyond the physical and is more integrative because everything is connected.

Soon after I graduated with my bachelor's I worked as a personal trainer at Equinox Fitness in Miami, FL. There, too, I noticed a common theme with the clients I got to work with who experienced body aches and pain (especially back pain), who were overworked, highly stressed, always on the go, feeling the need to hustle and stuck in the do-ing all day. They experienced poor sleeping habits, and were unaware of how their thoughts, words, and lifestyle choices were affecting how they felt and performed in life. I gained further insight into how emotions influenced the way the body moved. And the clients who were more in tune, aware, and conscious with their body, thoughts, and daily choices that felt nourishing and supportive, performed better in all aspects of their life: Career, relationships, connection to Self and others.

Clients came to me in hopes of losing weight to look and feel better. They wanted to manage their stress with movement and desired to sleep better and experience a healthier life. Yet, they felt the need to punish their body with beliefs that their body was ugly, broken, and not good enough. So, they believed working out and lifting weights could solve the perceived issues. Training and working out can be supportive, but if the heart, if all matters of the heart are not tended to, you can only go so far before you burn out.

And yes, I, too, experienced this burnout.

For 15 years, I connected with patients and clients who desired the same thing: freedom – freedom from pain and emotional stress. And I learned they were mirrors for me. They reflected to me, that I, too, was energetically, physically, mentally, spiritually, and emotionally malnourished. I, too, perceived my body as ugly, broken, and not good enough. I, too, judged and shamed myself. I, too, struggled with feeling the need to hustle and go-go-go all the time, and I experienced burnout more than once.

Why?

Because I was programmed to believe that working all the time to pay bills is the way to live a 'successful' life. Slowing down was a sign of weakness. Suppressing emotions was learned and normalized. I was fuelled by the need to over perform and seek external validation. And I was afraid of failing.

Fear of failure relates to believing you're not good enough. Fear of failure relates to forgetting who you are. Fear of failure is an illusion, a perception limiting your true potential.

Failure doesn't exist. Learning does.

Perceived failure originates from shame, guilt, deception, and the need to control, manipulate, and suppress one's true potential. One cannot fail for it doesn't exist. Believing in Self overpowers perceived failure. Loving the Self dissolves it.

Why does doing, hustling, and feeling the need to go-go-go lead to pain, aches, injuries, body shame, and burnout?

The right hemisphere of the brain influences the left side of the body. The right hemisphere is the Feminine/Mother energy (the creative side) and relates to flow and ease, heart connection, a space of receiving, receptivity, and accepting life as is.

The left hemisphere of the brain influences the right side of the body. The left hemisphere is the Masculine/Father energy (the analytical/logical side) and relates to self-confidence, courage, strength, conscious productivity, and being proactive by choosing inspired actions, and feeling present in every now moment.

The common theme with myself, patients, and clients was an imbalance between the do-ing and be-ing, the giving and receiving, the Masculine and Feminine energies, and uncaring of Self: mind, heart, body, and spirit.

For over a decade, I felt stuck in the go-go-go.

I always felt the need to *do* to get things done because I was afraid of what would happen if I were to stop. I was afraid of feeling all of the suppressed emotions. I was afraid of meeting myself wholeheartedly.

I admit, the going and doing mind-set led me very far: accepted into physical therapy school in California after four years of rejection from numerous schools, earned a doctorate in physical therapy with high honours at the age of 29, transitioned from working at outpatient clinics to working independently as a sole practitioner four years after graduating, received certifications in all things related to the body, movement, functional medicine, energy healing, and more. And yes, I'm grateful for it all.

But the constant going and doing wasn't sustainable because it affected my performance with how I was showing up for myself and others.

So, how did I shift from dissonance to resonance, from burnout to sustenance, and harmonise with the energies?

I connected within.

I travelled through time while lying on the floor with my eyes closed.

I was shown moments of my life when I was younger, disliking my body, feeling unhappy, and not knowing how to connect to myself in a way that felt soothing, loving and nourishing.

I did the complete opposite for a long time and then wondered why I was experiencing physical pain, health issues, and body shame.

So, I tended to younger Sofia, and held her and told her 'I love you' because at the end of the day, that's all I needed.

All I was craving for was love.

Then another moment from the past flashed next, and again, I held younger Sofia and told her that I loved her. One moment after another, until I was led into the present moment and I expressed out loud...

I LOVE EVERY SINGLE PART OF ME.
I LOVE EVERY SINGLE PART OF ME.
I LOVE EVERY SINGLE PART OF ME.

All parts.

The shadows: Fear, self-doubt, anxiety, anger, AND the light: courage, grace, beauty, and love that I AM.

Every single part because fear brings love, doubt brings courage, shame brings compassion.

It's all needed to heal, grow, evolve, ascend, and rise in love.

Rise in love with myself first.

So, I celebrate today (and everyday) that I get to live, breathe, and say, "I love every single part of me."

Do-ing is an outward energy, action-oriented (Masculine energy).

Be-ing is an inward energy, receptive-oriented (Feminine energy).

When the doing and being are out-of-harmony, it can lead to burnout, pain, self-doubt, and you feel disempowered, unsupported, confused and lost – all the things that don't allow you to feel your best.

When in-harmony, you feel more present, calm, confident, and connected.

Doing and being are the ebbs and flow of life.

You can't have one without the other.

Action, rest.

Life, death.

Yin, Yang.

Dark, light.

Moon, Sun

Sound, silence.

Feminine energy, Masculine energy.

Right brain hemisphere, Left brain hemisphere.

Inhalation, exhalation.

They co-exist for a divine reason.

I am present and accept life as is unites the sacredness of the Masculine and Feminine energies.

'Present' is sacred action. 'Accept' is sacred receptivity – which means you receive life here and now.

I am present and accept life as is. My heart is open to receiving life here and now are expressions of Sacred Union.

Sacred Union is a joining, a coming together from the heart – pure, untethered like water, when in harmony with flow, the flow of being, existing, living, accepting life as is wholeheartedly. Sacred Union is a giving and receiving of divine unconditional love from the inside-out.

The Divine Path of Life is not about the job, credentials, or money. The Divine Path of Life is about coming home to your heart so you can unite with the sacredness deep inside, unite with unconditional love, unite with your power and the truth of who you are and why you're here; and unite with the creative life force inside you.

Wholehearted receiving, wholehearted giving – from the essence of your presence – is sovereignty, a reclamation, a returning of true nature.

I am present and accept life as is.
My heart is open to receiving life here and now.

And the design of your body harmonises the co-existence of sacred action and receptivity when energetically, spiritually, physically, mentally, and emotionally nourished from the inside-out.

The central nervous system includes the sympathetic nervous system (fight-or-flight) and the parasympathetic nervous system (rest-digest-rejuvenate). The sympathetic nervous system supports the body when needing to escape a life-threatening situation. The blood vessels in the digestive tract constrict so that the blood can circulate to the muscles for you to run/move your body away from danger. Internal and external stress heightens the sympathetic nervous system, and when in this state for prolonged periods of time, the body enters a catabolic (breakdown) state.

The parasympathetic nervous system supports the body with rest, rejuvenation, repair, and digestion without you needing to effort. The nerve that is prominent/active in this state is the vagus nerve. The vagus nerve is the tenth cranial nerve (CN X) and is the longest cranial nerve of the body originating in the brain then travels down the throat towards your lungs, heart, digestive tract (stomach and intestines), spleen, liver, and kidneys. The vagus nerve connects to the three brains (brain, heart, gut), and shares an energetic communication between all three.

Stress disrupts the function of the vagus nerve predisposing you to digestive issues, brain fog, fatigue, emotional distress, and anything that's not in alignment with rest, rejuvenation, healing, and harmony.

Intentional breathing is a simple solution to support the vagus nerve and harmonise the connection within (to receive more strategies that support the vagus nerve, check out my first book *The End of Back Pain: The Secret to Gaining Relief and Staying Active)*.

Being aware of longer exhalation throughout the day allows your body to feel calmer and more present. Intend your exhalation to breathe out all tension, worries, fear, and discomfort. And intend your inhalation to breathe in peace, love, healing, light, connection, and freedom.

When your body feels safe, supported, and calm, your heart gets to speak and express what she needs.

A message from your heart...

Do you feel free?

Do you feel free when you don't express your authentic self? When you suppress emotions?

Do you feel free when you feel love for someone yet don't tell them? When you feel grateful for their presence, yet don't express it?

Do you feel free when you avoid connecting to your body and supporting it with what it needs? When you don't ask me what the pain means so you can receive the gift and medicine?

Do you feel free when you allow the thoughts of worry and anxiety to rule your day? When you forget that I'm here to support you in every way?

Do you feel free when you create bricks of shame, guilt, resentment, and heartache inside of you? When you build walls so I can't experience divine unconditional love?

Do you feel free?

Because I don't.

I'm here, yet you choose to dismiss me when I whisper, "I need you." When I sing my song of desires, yet you choose to not listen.

To feel free begins with connecting to me.

I have everything you need: Love, wisdom, healing, and all that you're worthy of receiving.

I'm here, ready to embrace you and welcome you in.

It's okay. You're safe to feel me.

So, breathe out, clear your mind, surrender, and journey within.

My love for you will set you free.

Love,

Your Heart.

Your body isn't broken. The connection to your body is. And it's not your fault because you've been programmed to believe that it is, and your cells have been programmed to believe your body is broken for generations. Now you get to shift that belief and recreate a new one, 'I love my body and my body loves me', so you can receive what you believe and perceive.

Chapter 4
Return to Love

Your heart is the first organ to be created and is worth connecting to.

When I was in physical therapy school, I got to hold a cadaver's heart in my hands for the first time and felt something electric happen deep inside me. An experience I'll forever remember.

The cells created the heart first for a reason. So, the heart *is* your first brain and is the prime communicator for the rest of your body. The signals, information, and messages your heart sends to the rest of your body are influenced by your thoughts, beliefs, and emotions. And what you're thinking and feeling extends beyond you several feet via your heart's electromagnetic field.

If you believe you're unworthy of receiving love, wealth, and prosperity, that vibration (energetic frequency) of unworthiness extends outside of you and magnetises people and events that mirror the belief of feeling unworthy.

If you believe you can't live a luxurious life because you don't have enough money, that belief vibrates beyond you and magnetises (attracts) people and events that mirror that belief over and over again until you choose to figure out why you have those beliefs, then shift that belief into an elevated one.

For example: Money is a healer, a lightworker shining light on how you perceive Her. Money has been blamed, shamed, and judged for many years. And the energy of blame, shame, and judgement has been circulating. Everything is energy. And energy is currency. Feeling afraid you'll lose money, run out, and never have enough spreads fear with every investment. 'Money is energy continuously flowing for me to heal, learn, and expand' is an energetic shift from lack to abundance. Energy cannot be destroyed, only transformed.

By recreating new beliefs and perspectives, your cells will begin to reprogram on a DNA level, and you begin to feel elevated emotions from the new beliefs and perspectives.

Joy, love, happiness, and vitality, are energies that expand you. And you get to spread expansive energies with every investment.

Everything you desire is already within you – it's all about remembering and choosing to heal, shift, and recreate elevated beliefs to live out a new story and spread love as your new currency.

Because you can and you get to.

I love myself!

I love myself in this very moment. I love who I am and nothing can remove the love I have for myself, for my inner child.

I love myself. I love myself. I love myself.

Money will no longer have power over me.

I love myself with and without money. My financial success doesn't ignite more love for myself. The love I have for myself in the present moment is my abundance, that's my wealth. My love for myself is rich – my love enriches my entire being.

My love for me is my abundance. That was the missing piece for me. And now I feel whole and complete. My love for me is my abundance. My love for me adds richness into my life. My love for me is my wealth!

That's the lesson. That's the medicine.

I had to feel the love for myself.

My love for me is my abundance!

And now I feel it in every single cell of my body!

This is my wisdom; this is my medicine.

My love for me is my abundance.

My love for me is my wealth.

My love for me is rich.

I feel everything transcending, transforming, shifting, reprogramming deep within me. Fears transmuting into self-love, deep self-love, abundant self-love.

This is it!

My love for me has been ignited.

That's my magic. That's my superpower – loving myself abundantly!

I lit a candle and closed my eyes and I immediately saw my ancestors cheering, celebrating that my love for myself set them free – set their spirit free from shackles.

We celebrated together in love and freedom.

Dancing around a bonfire, burning the shackles, transforming them into light and beauty. And we danced, we laughed, we smiled with so much joy in our hearts! I felt their spirits filled with so much excitement, and I felt it within myself too, celebrating with them, celebrating love and freedom.

Love heals.
Love sets us free.

Your cells have been carrying beliefs for generations. And it's up to you (divine responsibility) to dive deep, explore, and learn where your beliefs, perceptions, and lifestyle choices originate from.

It's a divine responsibility to dive in.

To me, responsibility means the ability to respond to Self and life with the awareness that everything and everyone reflects what's deep within you.

Divine responsibility allows you to pause and ask yourself, "What is this person/situation teaching me? What can I learn from this person/situation? Where in my life have I behaved/acted in a similar way? "How did I contribute to this conflict/argument?" What beliefs/fears am I holding onto? What aspects of my life am I blaming, shaming, judging?"

Doing so liberates your heart, mind, and body from carrying limiting beliefs and passing it onto generations after you. You choosing to know your Self on a deep cellular level allows you to heal and return to love – the energy of love begins by connecting to your heart, and your heart will spread the energy of love from the inside-out.

We need love to spread and be the new currency. The world needs more love and Heart-Earth connection so the world can unite as one.

Love is who I AM

In April 2021, I received a message about who I AM.

While meditating, I was shown an image with two spheres overlapping each other like a vertical Vesica Piscis sacred geometric pattern, and in the centre was the essence of who I AM.

The top sphere was GOD, the bottom sphere was MOTHER EARTH/GAIA, and in the middle connecting the two spheres was LOVE, the true essence, the core truth of who I AM. I was then guided on a perspective about love.

Love is our core frequency, our baseline, our foundation. We coexist because of love.

Love fuels our everyday living.

And you must connect to love when facing your shadows, lower vibrational frequencies such as anger, heartache, resentment, grief, guilt, and shame. And since every cell in our bodies contain information from generations before us, we get to acknowledge and feel the lower vibrational frequencies (emotions) without judgement and choose to heal ourselves by shifting the lower vibrational frequencies into higher vibrational frequencies such as forgiveness, gratitude, compassion, and acceptance with an awareness that your shadows are gold that need to be dusted off and cleansed. The shadows alchemize into gold when you open yourself to receiving the gifts, wisdom, and lessons the shadows served, and return to your true essence – which is love.

Every emotion is energy in motion and since energy cannot be destroyed, only transformed, we have the power to choose how every emotion serves us.

Emotions are superpowers opening portals into the past so lower vibrational energies can be alchemized into divine unconditional love, and a potential future is created in the here and now. Emotions create reality. Emotions, when felt from the heart, can transform into gold, and offer infinite possibilities and opportunities for expansive growth.

Remember, everything is with purpose on purpose – the design of your body, the experiences of your life, every moment, every person you cross paths with, everything (just like your cells), serve a purpose for you to heal, learn, grow, and evolve as a person, a human being desiring to 'be', breathe, and experience life with more connection and vitality.

So many moments in one day from sunrise to sunset.

One can feel and experience moments that alter time and space.

Moments that change your life. Moments that lead you towards your truth, your true essence, in the raw. Moments opening your heart to be vulnerable, to lean into vulnerability and feel it break you open, tear you apart, to reveal the light, the silence, the pause of wisdom.

Moments filled with memories and stories that can be rewritten and transformed on a DNA level for you to no longer need to carry the hurt anymore; no longer need to carry the extra weight it had on you because the moments are there to be reflected upon, to learn, to grow, to remember where you came from, where you've been, how far you've come so you can appreciate the now.

And the now is where all the moments can be felt and experienced to create the future you want – a future filled with whatever you want to fill it up with as you fill yourself up first with moments that open your heart, break you open, tear you apart, to reveal your light in the raw, in the vulnerable rawness.

And from this rawness you grow a new skin – a skin of love, strength, courage, and abundance – all with gratitude – gratitude towards all the moments felt and experienced from sunrise to sunset.

To evolve into the person you desire to become, you must remember you are love because you can't evolve without love.

You can't even spell 'evolve' without the word 'love'.

And yes, it gets to be that simple.

Does it feel comfortable diving into yourself and facing all the thoughts, fears, beliefs, traumas, and emotions that have been avoided for so long?

No. It doesn't and that's okay.

You can lean into the discomfort and allow the process to unfold at your pace.

So, every lower vibrational frequency (emotion, thought, belief) serves a purpose and you get to choose how it can serve you. Anger can be transformed into understanding, acceptance, and forgiveness. Grief can be transformed into letting go, surrender, and being present. Shame can be transformed into freedom. And to feel the lower vibrational frequencies, you must pause and create space for it all to come up to the surface.

Invitation

Whenever you feel angry, frustrated, ashamed, unsupported, and unloved, place one hand over your heart and the other below your belly button, breathe out and connect to Mother Gaia. Pause. And feel into the uncomfortable emotion fully. Connect to the area of your body where it hurts and aches.

Exhale. Breathe it out.

Then ask your heart, "What do I need healing from?" Pause and listen. Listen to your heart. The heart that's made of many cells. The heart that shares the same frequency as Mother Earth (heart and Earth share the same letters too)!

The heart that is connected to all. Connect to her and listen. Then ask, "What's the gift in this? What's the gift in this discomfort? What is this person/situation/moment teaching me?"

Because everything is a reflection of the cells within you.

Your inner world reflects onto your outer world and vice versa. And to create a better outer world, you must heal and love your inner world.

When you discover the gift, the lesson and wisdom, that becomes your medicine. And that medicine returns you back to love, the vibration of love, the true essence of who you are.

Love overrides fear every single time.

Love fuels the spirit of your heart to alchemise darkness into light.

Choose love and let love choose you daily.

Kate's Journey

What was the divine catalyst in your life for you to know yourself on a deeper level and reclaim your self-worth?

I have the most amazing husband on the entire planet. He is so beautiful, kind, generous, supportive, and hysterically funny! Every day I feel honoured to be able to share this earthly journey with him. The way he sees me is the way I have always wished I could see myself. Having such a close partner allowed me to have deep conversations about how and why he sees me in a certain light and for me to be able to articulate why I didn't see myself the same way. Over time he would remind me, "When you walk into a room the entire mood shifts...in a good way, but sometimes not so good."

My standard response: "I didn't do anything. I walked in." I began to notice that the times when I was shifting the room in a 'not so good way' were the times when I wasn't really present in the moment, or I didn't really want to be there. I wasn't upset about being in the room, I just didn't care. It came off as 'bad vibes'. At the same time, it felt powerful to be able to walk into a space and have people feel a shift in energy. He wasn't the first, or last, to tell me that. That 'power' to shift energy in a room felt overwhelming to me. Like I had to be happy every second for fear that someone else might think I was mad or that I might create bad vibes if I wasn't always thrilled about everything. How could I have such unintended power to shift vibration when I wasn't even trying?

I started law school in August of 2020, because I'd always wanted to go and Covid really helped me pivot. Again, I was getting messages from other students and professors about my powerful, inspirational presence – we were on ZOOM!! Again, overwhelmed. In my second year of law school, I reached out to a woman in LA, originally from the UK, who is a celestial healer, guide and Reiki Master. For my birthday I gifted myself a one-on-one session with her. Our first session was so meaningful and impactful. She said, "Angel Uriel is lifting the veils of illusion to break false beliefs about yourself and old conditions." I sat with it and tried to meditate on it (as much as my ADHD would allow) and did some reflection. In February of 2022 I decided to reach out to her again and join her celestial tribe which allowed me monthly one-on-one sessions with her. I had this dream to study at Pepperdine Law School for a few weeks and she helped me manifest a place to stay, money to pay tuition and the ability to take the time off and go.

In June of 2022, on my last day of class at Pepperdine, I was participating in a negotiation session designed and facilitated by four women in my class who I had come to adore. They were rising 2L's (meaning they had just finished their first year of law school) but they were so intelligent and funny, super endearing and I loved seeing them every day. The negotiation had me and another student, an actual lawyer, negotiating for a job at his 'firm'. My fact pattern said that I was highly educated, had many accolades, and gave an average salary for the market. There was no negotiation. I said I need $85,000 per year, he said 'okay' and we were done. I was proud of myself for asking for $10k over the average market salary. When we finished the exercise, he showed me his fact pattern which said, "You'll pay between $85,000 up to $105,000, it doesn't matter to you what the number is." I started sweating, shaking, and had to leave the room to burst into tears in the bathroom. I was shocked by my own reaction.

The women who designed the question all came into the bathroom immediately to check on me. The 'baller' of the group said, "I gave you that question because you are such a baller!"

Another one said, "You are so impressive!"

I cried harder and out poured these words: "No matter how much I do, how many degrees I have, how many certifications, how much experience, it's never enough. I feel I deserve more, and I always settle for less because I don't want anyone to think I'm taking advantage of the situation."

I say, "Take what you can get and maybe next time someone will see your value."

I typed a thank you text to them on the plane on the way home and waited to send it until I felt better. I briefly fell asleep on the plane and clearly heard, "Why are you mad at the person who accepts the number you give them? They *see* your worth, you don't." I started sweating again and was in a panic to get the plane on the ground so I could send the women my text, get home and try to release the anxiety that was building to epic proportions. I spent several days carefully crafting an email to my healer about my reaction in class, not feeling worthy, knowing better and not being able to separate the logical from the emotional. We agreed to start some ancestral healing in our next session.

Before that occurred, I got a text from my dear friend Dr Sofia Costa asking if I had time for a Facetime chat to catch up on all things. One June 30, 2022, we had a four-hour chat where we talked, channelled, cleared out and reclaimed our power and self-worth just by sharing our experiences. Just talking about my experience and how it paralleled some of her own experiences and past experiences we had together was so healing. That wasn't even our plan! The literal second her face came up on my screen my entire body started tingling and we immediately connected, and words came pouring out of us both.

Upon reflection, I realise that moment in the law school bathroom sobbing in front of four virtual strangers, who at that point I would have traded places within a heartbeat, saw what my husband sees. They saw what others see and convey to me, but I failed to understand and accept. They barely knew me and they saw in me what I refused to believe thinking that those things made me 'egotistical'. That one 'baller' who, when I first saw her, made me think, *If I were in my early 20s with that swagger I could take over the fucking world*, wasn't showing me that I was a fraud, I was not an imposter. She was showing me a mirror. It was in that moment that I decided that I was not going to let her, or anyone else down by not standing in my power and taking responsibility for what I put out into the world knowing that what will come back is more than I hoped for because I finally connected to the divine within instead of looking for answers outside of myself.

Chapter 5
Everything Is Energy

You are what you eat, absorb, and can't eliminate (let go). And the Universe responds to what you eat, absorb, and can't eliminate (let go).

And it's not just with food – it's your thoughts, beliefs, fears, and emotions too. Just like your skin sheds dead skin cells daily, you, too, need to shed, purge, release, and detox from thoughts, beliefs, fears, and emotions that are not an energetic match for the reality you desire to experience. Whether your heart desires vitality, longevity, a stronger body, a conscious relationship, wealth, abundance, prosperity, connection, a supportive community, luxurious living – it's all energy.

The entire essence of *you* is energy.

You're an electric, cosmic, powerful multi-dimensional being of light with energy flowing through you and around you. You're the creator of your reality. And you have the power to shift energy with thoughts, words, and intentional actions.

"We are quite literally beings of light, each radiating a very vital life force and expressing an actual light field around our bodies – the totality of each cell expressing and contributing to a vital field of light that carries a message." – Dr Joe Dispenza, *Becoming Supernatural: How Common People are doing the Uncommon.*

You are a dynamic sphere, an all-encompassing sphere with sacred geometric patterns and chemical reactions fuelled by the energies of light and sound, frequencies of thoughts and emotions, and vibrations from your daily choices and intentions – co-creating a unique resonance that pulsates from deep within you. Your body encompasses spinning wheels of energy centres called chakras. There are seven main energy centres that carry information and correspond with different areas of your body, organs, systems, meridians, emotions, and beliefs. Every chakra is an energy of light, unique with its own sound, frequency, colour, element, and sacred geometric pattern. When you experience stress/trauma (sympathetic nervous system response), the energy centres are disrupted, affecting the flow of energy throughout your body.

The Complete Guide to Chakras authored by April Pfender is a great resource to gain further insight into each chakra (there are plenty of resources out there, so I encourage you to connect to the ones that resonate most with you).

Here is a brief outline of the seven main chakras, including their associated elevated beliefs and emotions:

Root Chakra
Colour: Red
Musical Note: C
Element: Earth
Body Location: Base of spine, sacrum, hip/pelvis, sex organs, intestines, colon, bladder, rectum, legs, feet.

Root chakra relates to foundation, the ability to provide for oneself, feeling safe and secure in your body and environment, feeling physically, emotionally, and financially supported, and relates to primal instincts.

Sacral Chakra
Colour: Orange
Musical Note: D
Element: Water
Body Location: 1–2 inches below belly button, sacrum, hip/pelvis, lower abdomen, womb space, sex organs, kidneys, bladder, intestines, lower back.

Sacral chakra relates to creativity, passion, inspiration, sensuality, pleasure, and a sense of belonging and intimacy.

Solar Plexus
Colour: Yellow
Musical Note: E
Element: Fire
Body Location: Base of sternum and above belly button, midback, upper digestive system, stomach, liver, gallbladder, small intestines, spleen, pancreas, diaphragm, upper abdomen, lower oesophagus.

Solar plexus relates to personal power, clarity with purpose and sense of self, sovereignty, confidence, vitality, and the ability to perceive obstacles as opportunities.

Heart Chakra

Colour: Green

Musical Note: F

Element: Air

Body Location: Centre of chest, respiratory and circulatory system, diaphragm, oesophagus, heart, thymus, lungs, breasts, shoulders, arms, hands.

Heart chakra relates to the connection to self, divine unconditional love, happiness, empathy, compassion, purity, acceptance, and the bridge between Heaven and Earth.

Throat Chakra

Colour: Blue

Musical Note: G

Element: None

Body Location: Base of throat, neck, ears, jaw, mouth, teeth, vocal cords, trachea, thyroid glands, parathyroid glands, upper oesophagus, cervical spine, shoulders.

Throat chakra relates to sound, expression, communication, listening to understand, decision-making, boundaries, discernment, speaking the truth and following your dreams.

Third Eye Chakra

Colour: Violet

Musical Note: A

Element: None

Body Location: The space between your eyebrows, eyes, parts of your brain, pineal gland, pituitary gland, hypothalamus, nose, and optic nerve.

Third Eye Chakra relates to self-reflection, insight on higher perspectives, 6th sense, intuition, clairvoyance, and telepathy; allows you to see the truth.

Crown Chakra
Colour: White
Musical Note: B
Element: None
Body Location: Top of head, skull, parts of brain, cerebral cortex, brain stem, pituitary gland, nervous system, and cranial nerves.

Crown Chakra relates to the divine connection with Spirit/Source/God, the bridge between you and the Universe, greater self-awareness, and higher vision that allows you to be present.

Emotions are energies in motion, and every chakra (energy centre) is associated with specific emotions, thought patterns, and beliefs. Whenever you feel stuck feeling a certain way or thinking the same racing thoughts, it's an opportunity to connect with the chakra associated with the elevated feeling/thought pattern you desire to experience so the energy can move and flow.

Your heart's desires are a higher vibration – an elevated energy – and to experience a higher vibrational life, you must eat thoughts and beliefs that empower you and support you; absorb love, abundance, joy, gratitude forgiveness, vitality, and prosperity daily; and eliminate (let go) fears, traumas, beliefs, and perceptions that are confining.

"The Elimination Diet: Remove anger, regret, resentment, guilt, blame and worry. Then, watch your life and health improve." – Charles F. Glassman.

'To cleanse' is what I heard during breath work.
Cleanse.
Shed the old.

So, what parts of me exactly?
What parts of me need to shed so I can grow?

Seeking validation.
Jealousy.
Doubting my power.
Not trusting my journey and seeking advice from someone else because I didn't think my intuition was strong enough or good enough.
Not feeling enough.
Feeling the need to lower my vibration, dim my light to make others comfortable.
Anxiety about the unknown, about the future.
Doubting who my beloved/soulmate is.
Self-doubt.
Not believing in myself, my power.
Forgetting who I am.
Acting out of obligation.
Weak boundaries.
Not allowing myself to express myself fully.
Holding back, playing small.
Blaming, shaming, judging.
Anger. Resentment.

Fear of not having enough money.

Feeling the need/urgency to post on social media to 'make it' in business.

Feeling afraid of others taking what I have.

Fear of how fast my life is changing.

People pleasing.

Giving my power away.

Fear of expanding.

Competitiveness, feeling the need to always be the best.

Perfectionism.

Fear of being judged.

Fear of not making the right decision; afraid of failing.

So, now, I release myself from my old Self.

I release her with love and grace.

I let her go.

I cut the cord and let her go.

And I reclaim all my power back to me and honour my divinity. I shed the old Self and embrace the new elevated version of me.

I am free.

I am free.

I am free.

To live and be the highest version most expansive divine me! Magnetic, vibrating at a higher frequency. And I can by trusting and being still – still in the present, allowing, receiving – because vibrating at a higher frequency, choosing to, is giving. I'm already giving with my frequency, divine frequency, the essence of my presence, and now I get to receive as I trust, breathe, in stillness, reclaiming and honouring my divinity.

So, why is this important?

Why is shedding, purging releasing, and detoxing yourself from fears, thoughts, beliefs, and emotions necessary as part of daily living?

So, you can create space for expansive experiences and opportunities, and receive miracles and blessings.

And remember the truth of who you are. Remembering who you are is the power of being known – a power of self-recognition. A power you can connect to now.

You are designed on purpose with purpose and it's time to live your life on purpose with purpose. You are deserving of it all. You are worth experiencing the richness of life from the inside-out. And your heart's desires need to be expressed, shared, trusting it's all possible for you – everything is.

And it begins by *believing* that your heart's desires exist now – not yesterday or tomorrow. *Now.*

Your heart's desires exist now because of your existence.

Believe it's all within you. The energy you wish to feel and experience daily exists inside of you. Believe. Choose to turn the light switch on. Feel your desires, your future life happening right now within you. No need to worry about the details of how it's going to work out. Let go, surrender, and rest in the Universe's actions.

Fear influences beliefs and perceptions to limit and confine. And fear is a by-product of an experience, a trauma, and a by-product of forgetting who you are.

Fear blinds you, covering your eyes with a veil of deception and lies. Fear is an entity keeping you in the dark, paralyzing your nervous system from expanding in your light.

And at the same time, fear is needed. Fear co-exists with love. Fear is a catalyst for you to remember the power within you and wake up – wake up to the truth that you are love. You are the breath of life, the heartbeat of the Universe, inhaling and exhaling in cosmic rhythm with the Divine.

So, yes, acknowledge the fears you feel and experience because fear serves a purpose guiding you to choose love and live out a new belief that expands your light, frees your Spirit, and opens your heart to receive blessings.

Heart-Earth Connection

Your blood shares the same minerals and elements as the Earth and stars. And your heart and brain share the same frequency as the Earth. The frequency is called Schumann Resonance measured at 7.83 Hz.

You, Earth, and the stars co-exist together for a reason.

It's all connected.

We are all connected.

When you heal, the Earth heals. When the Earth heals, you heal.

The experience is a divine partnership – a sacred reciprocity.

Earth and heart even share the same letters. The answer and solution are written there in front of you – when you connect to your heart, you connect to the Earth. And when you connect to the Earth by spending more time in nature, gardening, grounding, hiking, going to the beach, mountains, jungles and forests, and by eating food designed by Mother Nature, you deepen the connection to your heart and body. Plants, trees, fruits, vegetables, herbs, and flowers hold medicinal powers. Sprouting from the darkness of soil, absorbing water from the snow and rain, and rising to receive the light from the moon and sun, they carry a life force that can nourish our bodies and spirit.

Your breath is also connected to Earth.

Every time you exhale, carbon dioxide (CO_2) is released. The trees, plants, herbs, and flowers then use the CO_2 as fuel for photosynthesis to produce oxygen (O_2) for you to breathe in. And the most important phase of breathing is the exhalation phase. Your exhalation brings life to Earth's creations. And you receive life from Earth's creations.

The point of sharing all of this is to open your awareness that your body is beyond physical, and you're divinely connected to everything and everyone around you. I understand it's easy to forget when you experience pain, stress, overwhelm, and doubt why you exist in the first place.

You feel drained, tired, burned out and fragmented attempting to do everything all at once, and allow urgency and the need to control outcomes to overpower you. And to be honest, it doesn't even feel good in my body at the moment as I'm describing how it feels when we forget how divinely connected we are and the power we hold within us.

So, let's pause for a minute.

Take a deep breath into your heart and body. Then exhale all the air out. Repeat two more times.

Okay, I feel more grounded and at ease now, which I feel you do too.

So, returning to remembering that you are divinely connected to everything and everyone.

Your body *is* Earth, stars, light, and energy.

You are a human being.

You are of the Earth to be in God.

That's what 'human being' translates to. The word 'human' comes from the Latin word 'humus' which means 'Earth' and the word 'being' when broken up into Be-In-G – the letter 'G' to me represents God. 'Be' means to live, breathe, exist, and connect to the essence of 'I AM.'

You are a human being.

You are of the Earth to Be in God.

Live in God. Breathe in God. Exist in God.

As a human being, you are of the Earth to be in God within. 'To be in' is the act of seeing, listening, feeling, loving, and supporting your Self wholeheartedly; an act of receiving your Self in totality.

And the omnipresent, expansive energy of God/Love resides in your heart.

God is the embodiment of Love.
Love is the embodiment of God.

You are of the Earth to Be in God so you can see the I AM within your heart.

Your body is cosmic, intelligent, electrical – a powerful source of energy that can create anything and heal itself. And it's supported by the Earth and stars – so the more you connect to nature's elements, the more connected you'll feel with the energy of God/Love within your heart.

My Visit to the Happiest Country in the World

I choose to connect with Mother Earth and integrate Her wisdom daily. Honouring my body honours the Earth and my lineage. And I've witnessed the healing people get to experience and the happiness they exude when they choose to honour their body, the land, and their ancestors' traditions of living simply.

In March 2017, I was invited by a friend to travel to Bhutan, a country recognised as one of the happiest in the world. During my ten days of exploring the beautiful country with a group and tour guide, I got to experience and witness the locals' way of living. They value happiness, connection, sustainability, and acknowledge suffering as part of one's journey towards enlightenment. They respect each other and the land they steward, co-existing in harmony as a community. The country measures gross national happiness and focuses on the people's health and vitality over how much money they're making. The passing on of ancient wisdom, ceremonies, and traditions keeps their culture alive for generations.

One of the adventures during the trip was a visit to a school where children get to create art with their hands in 13 different ways. Painting, wood carving, clay sculpting, masonry, paper making, wood turning, embroidery, hand weaving, and blacksmithing are some examples of ancient practices that have been passed on for generations.

This quote was painted on the wall of the school building we visited:

"Get skilled. Be somebody! Be useful to yourself. Be useful to your parents. Be useful to community. Be useful to Tsa-Wa-Sum."

The tour guide led us into every room of the school and we got to witness the children use their hands to create. Every child creating looked focused and present without cell phones or any type of electronics nearby.

'Art' is embedded in the word 'heart'.

And your hands are an extension of your heart which means handcrafted creations are infused with light-filled heart energy. Creating with your hands is an enlightening experience and sharing your creation spreads light, love, and beauty. I got to witness first-hand the power of handcrafted creations when I observed my mother paint, sew, and design the house with heart-opening décor. She inspired my sisters and I to paint and create – a meditative practice we continue to integrate.

I'm grateful I got to experience Bhutan's magic. I definitely took notes from the local natives on what living simply looks like and feels like, and let me tell you, it was an enlightening experience.

The Natives and Indigenous are the first stewards of the land and are (and continue to be) the wisdom keepers of ancient practices that integrate the light and spirit. We must acknowledge their existence and support their sacred ceremonies to help restore Mother Earth and raise the consciousness of humanity.

"An ocean is a collection of drops, a rock is a collection of particles, but they are of equal value. The same is true for the love you have in your heart and mind." – Gyonpo Tshering, *The Bhutanese Guide to Happiness: 365 Proverbs from the World's Happiest Nation.*

It can be small, simple daily steps connecting to your heart and Earth. You choose whatever feels good to you. Remember, when you heal, Mother Earth heals. And when Mother Earth heals, you heal.

You're invited to deepen your Heart-Earth connection.

You can RSVP or you can decline too.

Your choice.

I am the New Earth (and so is every individual). So, when we each dive in to heal and become known, New Earth exists within you.

New Earth is an extension of you, an extension of your heart's frequency. Heal your Heart. Heal the Earth. Healing ourselves is co-creating the New Earth because we each evolve and ascend when we go deeper within, and we get to resonate at a higher frequency when we alchemise our fears and limiting belief systems that dimmed our light and lowered our frequency. The power of being known has greater purpose. The journey inward is for a reason, divine reason to get to know your Self, your truth, so the walls can come down and your heart can open to sing her song.

Sacred Water

Water flows bringing life to all creations.

Connected to the moon's gravitational pull, water takes up space on Earth and in our bodies too. She is the source of life nourishing us with ancient wisdom from the past and sustains us with her adaptability – shifting into three phases: Solid, liquid and gas.

An icosahedron sacred geometric pattern, fluid, rhythmic, abundant, sacred, and co-creator.

She's without limits, eternal. She doesn't grip onto anything or anyone. She flows without conditions or attachments. She is beauty, natural, and in the raw, reflecting the truth of who you are. She doesn't blame, shame, or judge.

Water is an element that co-exists within you and all around you. Water held space for the creation of you while in your mother's womb.

To not honour water as sacred means you don't honour yourself as sacred.

Without water, we are in a spiritual drought. To be honest, without water, we are in a drought in all ways (physically, mentally, and emotionally).

Our bodies are designed with 70–80% water – sustaining our entire system to flow, to be in flow, and provide support for us to be alive and live this life and experience every moment. So, yes, water is sacred in the way its intelligence nourishes our spirit, vitality, our being and essence. We can honour the sacred water within us with our thoughts, words, and intentional actions. Water holds memories, remembering everything. The molecules of the water are influenced by the power of our energy – limiting beliefs, scarcity mind-set, the need to control fuelled by fear of the unknown creates dams within you, blocking flow, creating internal resistance and waves of emotions causing stress and turbulence. Water is sacred and we are made of water for a reason.

Earth is made of water too, reflecting the sacredness we have within us. The oceans, lakes, rivers, creeks influence our brain and nervous system to feel more relaxed, receptive, and present.

"It's only recently that technology has enabled us to delve into the depths of the human brain and into the depths of the ocean. With those advancements our ability to study and understand the human mind has expanded to include a stream of new ideas about perception, emotions, empathy, creativity, health and healing, and our relationship with water. Several years ago, I came up with a name for this human-water connection: Blue Mind, a mildly meditative state characterized by calm, peacefulness, unity, and a sense of general happiness and satisfaction with life in the moment." – Wallace Nichols, *Blue Mind: The Surprising Science That Shows How Being Near, In, On, or Under Water Can Make You Happier, Healthier, More Connected, and Better at What You Do.*

Honouring the sacred water within you, honours the sacred waters outside of you and vice versa. Honour with thoughts, words, awareness, intentional actions to consciously nourish your cells (self). For us humans are energetic beings, fuelled by light and electricity.

And what fuels light and electricity?

Flow.

Water flow.

Water is nourishment for the mind, body, heart and soul. To not honour the sacredness of water within you and around you with thoughts, words, and intentional actions creates dams blocking you from experiencing the richness of life from deep inside. And instead, a life of drought is a result when water isn't honoured and supported as an essential element to feel abundant and alive.

My love and respect for water began at a young age. Born on the island of Puerto Rico, I was surrounded by water. And when my family and I moved to South Texas, we went deep sea fishing often. My father taught my two sisters and me to respect and honour the ocean. Even on days when we didn't catch any fish, my father reminded us that we captured the beauty of the day and sea. He often expressed life lessons using the ocean as an example for us to connect to and relate.

For example, the waves of the ocean are like the moments of life you experience daily. You can't control the size of the wave nor the direction it's coming from. You can only accept the wave as is, learn from it, and admire the beauty each wave offers – which reminds me of one of my favourite quotes, "A smooth sea never made a skilled sailor." – Franklin Roosevelt.

Emotions are like the waves of the ocean. You can't avoid it. And you can't escape from it. The waves exist whether you like it or not. The more you resist feeling every wave of emotion, the greater the inner turbulence.

On July 16, 2010, a couple of my classmates from physical therapy school and I headed to the beach in Carlsbad, CA. It was only my sixth time out there in the ocean learning how to surf. With a borrowed wetsuit and surfboard, I was motivated to learn and experience the 'stoke' of catching a wave all the way to shore. As I was floating on the surfboard waiting for the next wave, I checked out my surroundings to see who was near us. My father taught my sisters and me at a young age to always check and assess your surroundings, and at the age of 17, I worked as a lifeguard at a water park on the beach.

As I was scanning and taking mental notes of the people near us in the ocean, I noticed a man with a large orange longboard. Moments later, I scanned the surroundings again and noticed the orange longboard, but this time, without the man. I cautiously waited for the man to appear, and after a while, I felt it was too long for a person not to appear. I let my classmates know I was going to swim out and check on him.

I felt a surge of adrenaline rush through every single cell of my body as I swam closer to the longboard afraid of what I was going to see. I found the man underwater, not moving and attached to the end of the surfboard leash. I immediately yelled at my classmates to get help and cried out to the surfers who were closer to help me. I grabbed the leash and pulled the man out of the water. I still remember what his face looked like as if the event happened yesterday: Purple, eyes closed, foaming at the nose and mouth – I honestly thought he was dead.

I treaded water holding his head up until a group of surfers and I worked together to place the man on a foam top longboard and float him to shore. By the time we made it to

82

shore, the paramedics were there waiting. My two classmates were also at the shoreline and embraced me when the shock of the experience hit me. As I was processing the events of what just happened, I was approached by a journalist who witnessed the event and asked if he could interview me. He recorded my response on his cell phone and later that day wrote an article titled 'Physical Therapy Student Saves Surfer's Life' on www.carlsbadistan.com.

As the paramedics were tending to the man who was saved and prepping him to be sent to the hospital, one of the man's friends who was out there surfing near him, approached me and asked me for my cell phone number. Several days later while I was studying for an exam, I received a phone call from an unknown number. Hesitant to answer, I pushed the green button to accept the call.

"Hi, is this Sofia Costa?"
"Yes."
"My name is Tony. You saved my life!"

Tears streamed down my face connecting to the man whom I thought wasn't going to make it.

A couple of days later, I got to meet Tony and several of his family members at the hospital. They shared that the doctors were impressed he survived because he had a seizure, and had he stayed underwater seconds longer, he would've died. He was 55 years of age at the time.

Several months later, I was awarded a Certificate of Amendment from the local police department. And Tony and I became friends – he even attended my graduation at the physical therapy school I was attending.

But what many didn't know was the internal turbulence of emotions I was feeling daily from the shock, trauma, and overwhelm of July 16, 2010. It hit me that there was something much bigger than me – otherwise, how did I know I needed to swim towards the orange longboard? What was guiding me? I asked so many questions trying to figure out why it all happened. And after deep self-reflection, I gained awareness that everything that ever happened in my life happened for a reason. From the day I was born with the umbilical cord wrapped around my neck to feeling the nudge to go to the ocean that day, I was led and guided every step of the way. Life is divinely orchestrated for a greater purpose, and there are no mistakes with the design of life.

I didn't enter the ocean for four years because the image of the Tony's face when I pulled him out of the water was imprinted in my memory. And every time my feet touched the ocean from the shoreline, a replay of the event happened every single time.

My nervous system would glitch out and my body relived the experience. My love for the ocean was paralyzed for four years. And I suppressed the emotions of the shock and trauma so that I can continue with my studies while attending physical therapy school. Seeing the ocean reminded me of the event–and it was as if every wave that came to shore was reminding me to connect with the waves of emotions within me so I can be cleansed and purified from the experience and learn from it. The ocean worked her magic and invited me to enter her world again.

Four years after the life-changing experience, I was working at a sports orthopaedic clinic in Santa Monica, CA and one of the patients I got to work with was a surfer recovering from an ACL repair surgery. He was young, vibrant, full of life, and was motivated to get back in the ocean and surf. After several weeks of intense rehab, he was ready to surf again. And I proposed the idea that I'll enter the ocean with him on his first day back to surf again.

He lent me one of his surfboards and we both paddled out past the break. He knew of the story of what happened back on July 16, 2010, and was supportive of me gradually returning to the ocean alongside him – both of us returning to her to overcome shock and trauma. The ocean welcomed us, wave after wave, nourishing us with her healing presence. And I got to witness the patient catch his first wave!

His joy and happiness spread out like a rippling effect, and I got to feel it too in every single cell of my body. From trauma to excitement, we were both liberated from what we were suppressing and afraid of feeling and facing.

The ocean infused us with medicine, strength, wisdom, and blessings.

I saved a life in the ocean and the ocean saved mine.

To continue with healing myself from feeling traumatised and afraid of the ocean, I decided to work with a surf coach for several weeks to support me with learning how to surf again and reignite my love for the ocean.

On the first day, I remember sitting on my surfboard, floating in the water, waiting for a wave when my surf coach said, "You're not going to catch anything today with all the emotional baggage you're carrying."

I immediately felt triggered hearing his words. I barely knew the guy and he was already expressing the truth. And to be honest, he was right. I didn't catch a single wave that day. And that triggering sentence changed me in a way I didn't even think it could. That triggering sentence was the healing I needed. It wasn't about catching waves, it was about feeling the waves inside of me and learning to surf those with awareness, confidence, courage, and grace.

Every surf session thereafter, the coach had me focus on the heavy emotions I was still holding onto – anger, frustration, resentment – and use it as fuel to paddle, pop up, and surf.

Yes, I wiped out so many times and every time I did, he had me reflect on what happened, what did the wave teach me, and use the gained insight and wisdom to strengthen and support me for the next wave. The process felt intense and much needed for my healing because when I did surf a wave and felt the joy and excitement of the wave carrying me, feeling every emotion to experience the 'stoke' moment was well worth it.

He was a beacon of light for me and demonstrated what it looked like to honour the sacredness within you and around you. Before entering the ocean, he taught me to be intentional in a ceremonial way by offering a prayer of love and gratitude. We were entering her world, and purifying our hearts and spirit with love, intention, and gratitude was meaningful and important.

Water is sacred. And we must restore the sacredness of water with intentional thoughts, words, and actions.

"Since becoming entranced by the wondrous powers of water, I have been blessed with the opportunity to see and conduct experiments on many types of water from around the world. Each sample of water from a different part of the world has its own unique and beautiful characteristics.

I have also seen with my own eyes how the water of the world is becoming polluted. The World Trade Organization has stated that the twentieth century started with wars for oil, but that in the twenty-first century we will see wars for water.

Pollution originated within our own consciousness. We started to think that we wanted a bountiful and convenient lifestyle at any cost, and this selfishness led to the pollution of the environment that now affects every corner of the globe.

We have seen through the crystal photographs that water is the mirror of our souls." – Masuro Emoto, *The Hidden Messages in Water.*

Dr Masuro Emoto was an author and internationally renowned Japanese scientist who discovered the power of our own thoughts on water. He studied the changes of the molecular structure of water using words that were either lower in vibration or higher in vibration. And he found that the water molecules exposed to words that expressed love, gratitude, peace, and forgiveness transformed into a unique geometric shape that appeared like a crystalized snowflake. And when the water was exposed to images of war, anger, and hate, the molecule appeared to be disfigured and irregular in shape.

What would you like your water molecules to look like?

You can alchemise the water within your body, within your cells, and co-create a better reality for you to experience happiness and vitality.

Just like the moon influences the tides of the ocean, the moon in all her phases, influences the sacred water within you. Connect to your inner water by feeling every wave of emotion wholeheartedly and learn to love your Self in every phase of your heart-centred journey.

Hydrate with elevating thoughts, words, and intentional actions. Connect to love and gratitude before sipping water, organic coffee, or tea from a glass and before taking a shower or bath.

And be in flow with every life's moment.

Sound Healing

Believe it or not, you're a sound healer.

We all are.

The beat of your heart creates sound, the tone of your voice, the sound of your words, the vibration of your presence, the note of your soul, all unique and healing when you're in harmony with your Self – heart, mind, body – and in harmony with the world.

Your choice of words creates a sentence that can sound like a beautiful melody, or it can sound rough, harsh, and aggressive. Your sound is unique, and you have the power to conduct your own orchestra with your thoughts, words, intentions, and emotions. Your song can heal, or it can hurt. Your choice. You're the conductor of your own inner orchestra. Low notes. High notes. All needed to play a symphony.

When I was young, I played classical piano for ten years. I performed at recitals and for five consecutive years, I participated in the Piano Guild Auditions. The Piano Guild

Auditions require you to memorise ten classical pieces and play it in front of a judge, one after the after, without knowing which piece you're going to be asked to play.

It was just me, the piano, and the judge in a room. The judge randomly chooses the piece, states the title and composer of the piece, then waits and listens. With confidence, presence, and my breath to calm my nervousness, my fingertips touched the piano keys and I immersed myself, recalling every note, every sound by memory. From heart to brain to hands, an energetic communication, creating harmony and flow with sound composed like poetry. A meditative experience – present, focused, and attentive with an open heart and clear mind connected to the magic of playing sound with every key I touched.

After playing every piece, I left the room and waited for the judge's rating and feedback on my overall performance. And I scored Excellent – the highest rating – every year! Now, do I remember any of those classical pieces today? Nope! But I got to experience the power of sound and discovered that what we are capable of as humans is limitless.

Once while playing the piano at a recital, I completely froze and forgot the entire middle section of the musical piece. Rather than running off the stage like how I've witnessed other kids do when they froze and forgot what to play next, I stayed on the piano bench and focused to remember and finish what I started.

In that moment of forgetting the middle section of the musical piece, I could feel my face getting hot from embarrassment and I attempted to play a couple of chords but the sound didn't feel right. So, I paused, took a deep breath and chose to keep going and play the last section of the piece that I remembered so I can finish playing the song. When I finished, I stood up, bowed in front of the audience and judges, and returned to my seat next to my parents. I told them I had forgotten an entire section of the piece and they didn't even notice! I received a high score and compliments from the judges because I chose to stay and finish what I started with grace and courage.

I learned then I had a choice: Rush off the stage because of fear, shame, and embarrassment or stay, connect to my breath and believe in myself.

And this experience relates to life. We all have a choice to decide what creates a better result that ignites our power, our light, our strength – even when you feel exposed, uncomfortable, vulnerable, and in the raw. You, too, can pause, take a deep breath, focus, and allow your heart to guide you.

Low notes.
High notes.
All needed to create the symphony of your life.

I stopped playing the piano when I went off to college. But music and sound continued to be a huge part of my life. Several years ago, I learned about sound frequency and how certain sound frequencies and musical notes correlate with your organs, chakras, and belief systems.

This wisdom of sound frequency has existed for thousands of years. Ancient civilizations understood the power of sound through chants, mantras, prayers, and toning. The power of sound can help heal the body because the vibration from sound waves penetrates through the body and creates energetic shifts on a deep cellular level that can support you with clearing and purifying.

In fall of 2020, I was drawn to play sound again after listening to an inner child guided meditation. During the meditation, I saw younger Sofia sitting on the sand along the shoreline. When I approached her, she looked sad. I asked her what she needed healing from and what she needed to feel better. "Sound," she said. "I want to play sound."

Several days later, I came across a self-guided online program to learn more about the history of sound healing and how to play various musical instruments like the crystal sound bowl.

During the program, I gained further insight about the Solfeggio frequencies, musical notes that correlate with each chakra, and how the world was first created by sound.

Each Solfeggio frequency correlates with an experience:

396 Hz – Liberation from fear.

417 Hz – When experiencing intense life changes.

432 Hz – Overall healing.

528 Hz – Miracles, DNA repair.

639 Hz – Harmonic relationships; improves connection.

741 Hz – Problem solving; enhance intuition.

852 Hz – Divine timing; Spiritual order.

963 Hz – Open third eye/pineal gland

You can play a Solfeggio frequency in the background while at home meditating, performing household chores, journaling, or while creating. You can tune in and listen anytime.

The first two musical instruments I invested in while going through the online sound healing program was the Tibetan Sound Bowl and a handcrafted rattle. As soon as I played the Tibetan Bowl for the first time, I felt my entire body wake up to the sound and resonance. It felt like sound was the missing link for my heart and spirit to further deepen and expand.

When I travelled to California in Fall 2021 to road trip from San Diego to Mt. Shasta, I found my first Alchemy Crystal Sound Bowl. Connecting with the powerful sound bowl activated my first instrument – my voice. I began harmonising, toning, and singing more than I ever had before. And I experienced deeper healing from the sound of the crystal bowls and from the sound of my voice.

As mentioned before, the parasympathetic nervous system is powered by the vagus nerve supporting you with rest, digestion, feeling calm, connected and present. Humming turns the vagus nerve on and shifts the energy of stress, worry, and overwhelm to peace and harmony here and now. Humming to yourself or a child nourishes the spirit of the heart.

Being is the sound of existence.

Invitation

Here is an invitation to activate your soul's note…

Close your eyes. Place both hands over your heart.

Breathe into your heart and allow the front and back of the heart to expand with every inhale.

Exhale any tension and anything else that's not allowing your heart to fully open.

Feel into your heart and notice what it feels like to connect to Her. Feel every beat.

Then connect to what the energy of love feels like. Notice where you feel the sensation of love in your body. Observe how you feel when you connect to the vibration of love. And allow the vibration of love to spread throughout your entire body. When you feel like your body has been filled with the vibration of love, hum or open your mouth and sing! Create an 'aaahhhh' sound from the space of love that you're in right now. Then create the sound 'om', the universal sound of creation. Feel the vibration from the sound of your voice. Allow the sound to flow through you. Allow the sound of love to travel from the inside-out.

"When we sing, we are orchestrating a breathing pattern in conjunction with the singing. It is based on the tempos of the song and the phrases sung. When we sing together, our hearts can entrain to similar patterns and can move to smooth, orderly, coherent heart rhythms and improve heart rate variability." – Barry Goldstein, *The Secret Language of the Heart: How to Use Music, Sound, and Vibration as Tools for Healing and Personal Transformation.*

You're a sound healer.

We all are.

Get to know your soul's note and sing your song to the Universe.

I was awakened around 4 a.m. – tossing and turning with thoughts and visions going through my head.

I tuned into a sound healing meditation and was immediately guided to my womb space where deeper shadows were hidden.

I cried feeling the darkness and allowed myself to let go and surrender.

My pelvic bowl, my pelvic sound bowl, received deeper healing.

The shadows are perceived fears blinding us from seeing through the lens of Divine Love clearly.

Fears hide the beauty that already exists deep within us.

Our inner light can shine and clear the path when we choose courage to walk The Path.

I am moving forward with love and courage in my heart. I allow the Universe to surprise me daily. And I'm grateful for everything as I continue to surrender and remember who I AM.

Part III
From 'Who Am I?' To I Am

Chapter 6
Generational Healing
Creates Generational Wealth

To know your Self on a cellular level means you're connected to the wisdom of your DNA.

Your DNA holds generations of wisdom, culture, tradition, traumas, and medicine for you to remember who are, where you come from, and share your legacy with the world. That's why you're worth knowing because your cells hold all the stories that are there waiting for you to connect to, experience, feel, and share.

To know yourself, you must dive in, journey inward, and explore the library of information within your cells. And when you do, when you decide to dive deeper into your Self, you heal, learn, grow, evolve, and liberate your ancestors from carrying the shame, guilt, and anger. You then get to connect to the wisdom of their experiences.

Choosing to heal your Self from beliefs and traumas that have been passed down generations, heals generations before and after you – and *that*, that decision of diving in, that choice, and commitment devoting yourself to the inner exploration of knowing *is* wealth.

You gain freedom. You experience a lightness deep within yourself, your heart, mind, and body. You no longer carry the heaviness and emotional baggage that has been passed on for so long. It's all free to go and can be alchemised when you decide, when you choose, to connect deeper and unlock your DNA's wisdom.

Genetic expression is not the only thing that gets passed down. Fears, beliefs, traumas, and wisdom too – all influencing your day-to-day living and behavioural patterns.

The fear of running out of money feels deep and has come up more than once for me.

It's generational fear from both sides of my family. Mother and Father since the beginning of time.

And it stops with me.

I no longer want to carry this fear and I no longer want my ancestors to carry it either. I don't want generations after me to continue to carry this fear of running out of money because it's time to trust that money is here to love us and support us to co-create and birth magic. We are here to serve Humanity to heal, grow, and evolve and shine light, our Divine Light, for the entire world to see the light within themselves, so they, too, can heal, grow, and evolve.

Divine Ancestors of Light, how do we get to heal ourselves from this fear of running out of money?

Because this fear has programmed us to hustle, overwork, over perform, burn out, not invest in ourselves, held us back from expanding and going bigger, dimmed our light and we played small for so long, we didn't allow ourselves to travel and explore the world, or share our gifts because we felt afraid it would cost too much, and if we had money, we felt scared it will be taken away, stolen; this fear of running out of money has held us back for too long and it's time to liberate ourselves so we can feel free to create, expand, evolve, shine our light, travel, explore, connect on a deeper level, share our gifts, birth magic, and live our lives luxuriously supporting each other.

Let's shift our belief and live out a new story.

Money is always circulating, like blood in our arteries and veins, it's always flowing in and out, in and out, like the waves of the ocean, and our breath. We breathe in and out. We are the breath of life, and our breath is love. Money is love and is always circulating. Nothing to fear. No need to fear anymore. We are safe to trust money is love and always circulating to serve ourselves and Humanity. Money spreads love because we are love. Fear of running out of money blocks the flow of money. Trust and believe money is always available for us to experience the richness of life because the energy of money is within us circulating like the blood in our arteries and veins. The energy of money is love, expanding us to evolve. Love circulates within us, continuously, because we are love. Love is our true essence and love never runs out.

Love is circulating within me now. And with this Divine Love circulating within me, I magnetize everything that is meant for me.

No need to chase.

No need to hustle for what I want.

No need to worry.

The love circulating within me magnetizes everything that is meant for me, meant for you, meant for the entire world.

The love circulating within me magnetizes everything for the greater good for all and it spreads beyond me.

And anything I invest in and co-create spreads Divine Love.

And so it is!

Inherited Beliefs

Beliefs are energies that get passed down generations. Your cells absorb everything which means what you think, feel, say, and believe impacts you on a DNA level.

How is that possible?

When your mother was being created in your grandmother's womb, your mother was already holding the eggs to create you. So, whatever your grandmother was experiencing during that time – whether she was experiencing depression, or any stressors, illness, traumas, thoughts/beliefs, and emotions, your mother absorbed it, and *you* absorbed it.

And when you were being created in your mother's womb, you absorbed everything your mother was feeling, believing, and experiencing too.

You not only inherit DNA and genetic expressions. You inherit beliefs, thoughts, stories, programs that have been passed down generations. So, if your ancestors were enslaved by fear and trauma, do you think they felt safe, loved, supported, and worthy?

Feelings of unworthiness are coming up right now at this moment, bringing tears to my eyes. My ancestors didn't feel worthy for the longest time – I imagine so after being enslaved by fear for generations.

Feelings of unworthiness are coming up – unworthy of love, unworthy of fame, unworthy of success, unworthy of money, and from this space, I don't feel safe with love, fame, success, and money.

To My Loving Ancestors,

Your worth has been embedded within you – it was never removed, it was never taken away – it may have felt like it – but your worth, your true worth is your spirit – and your spirit is unbreakable, resilient, strong and courageous. Your worth is love and love is your worth and all of it is your birth right. It's time to reclaim your worth, and continue to be. Recognising your own worth sets you free. Your presence is worthy in this world – even though it was dismissed and neglected – but you having honour within yourself, for yourself and for each other frees your spirit. Your worth is love, and love is your worth. Your worth is your wealth. Feeling worthy and recognising your worth, your value, your gifts, your magic is your wealth. You are all worthy and it's an honour to see and feel your worth. Your presence brings worth into this world. You are worthy to give and receive. I love you. You are loved. You are all loved.

The darkness is needed – it's there for us to dive into and feel – feel the aches, feel the grief, anger, resentment, heartache – feel and acknowledge, feel and understand, feel and receive its medicine, feel and honour it for it all serves its purpose.

Feeling sets you free – feeling sets your heart free – feeling sets your spirit free. Feeling creates flow within. Feeling brings harmony and peace. Feeling heals.

I was born in San Juan, Puerto Rico to a family of artists, healers, shamans, medicine men and women. My mother is from San German and my father is from San Juan. My parents inspired me to live a wholehearted life so I can co-create a new paradigm. Connecting with family and listening to their stories allowed me to gain a deeper understanding about my lineage.

Puerto Ricans are an ancestral blend of three races: Spanish, African, and Taíno Native.

The Taíno Natives of Puerto Rico were killed, persecuted, raped, neglected, and forced to alter their way of living. Families were separated, land and resources were stolen, their wisdom and spiritual practices were taken advantage of, and disease spread among them.

I felt anger towards the colonizers, and blamed, shamed, and judged their catastrophic actions. I felt heartache and pain for the Africans and Natives.

Holding onto anger, heartache, and pain resisted love and forgiveness. I chose to let go and release myself from the heaviness. I can't change what happened in the past, but I can shift the energy. I decided to shift my perspective and see the past through the lens of love and compassion. I gained clarity, courage, strength, and insight. And I forgave myself for blaming, shaming, and judging for so long. I forgave the colonizers, Africans, and Natives. Forgiveness liberated my heart from generational fear and trauma.

Forgiveness sets you free from gripping onto the past. Forgiveness is the greatest act of self-love because you open your heart to meet your Self and tend to the pain you were holding onto for so long.

Forgive yourself for blaming, shaming, judging yourself.

Forgive others for blaming, shaming, judging you.
Forgive your family.
Forgive your ancestors.
And set yourself and ancestors free.

The past needs to be acknowledged with an open heart and awareness so a better future is created.

During the pandemic lockdown in 2020, I received a divine message while I was sleeping: 'Ancestral healing. The world needs ancestral healing', and I was being nudged by spirit to talk about it and share on social media during that time. I felt intimidated and immediately said 'no way' because I feared I would be judged, dismissed, and blamed. Who am I to talk about ancestral healing?

But who am I not to?

So, I connected with my ancestors and dove deeper than ever before. I began reading a book my uncle gifted I called *Taínos and Caribs: The Aboriginal Cultures of the Antilles* authored by Sebastian Robiou Lamarche. I learned about Taíno culture, their way of life, traditions, and stories they believed in.

Every village had a shaman that integrated plant medicine to see, feel, and hear messages from Great Spirit about the stars and cosmos, specific flowers and herbs to use when treating illnesses and injuries, future wars and conflict to prepare for, where to grow food and when to harvest according to the lunar phases and weather – ancient wisdom divinely channelled by the shaman and shared with the chief to support the village.

Ancient wisdom is in my DNA too. And I continue to learn about my heritage.

I forgive the past. I forgive my ancestors. I forgive with gratitude for the experiences because it all happened for a reason.

And I choose to alchemize the pain and awaken the power of love within me so I can be the legacy of love the world is needing.

You inherit beliefs, fear, heartache, and trauma. You inherit ancient wisdom and cosmic intelligence.

Remember, it's not only what you absorbed in your mother's womb, but also what your mother absorbed in her mother's womb and so on. Even what your father lineage experienced, you inherited too.

Dive into *you*. And understand that what you're experiencing and feeling in the present moment is not just from you. It's from generational patterns that have led you to where you are today. You have the power to transform inherited beliefs and generational trauma by forgiving what happened in the past so you can receive, wisdom, healing, and heart medicine for yourself and family lineage.

Generational healing creates generational wealth.

Wealth is love and freedom.

Be the legacy of love the world is needing.

Heal the We

During Holy Fire Reiki III Master Training in May 2021, the teacher/mentor guided the group on a meditation. A journey where I was led to a waterfall. I saw myself sitting on a large rock with the waterfall to the left of me and the flowing water moving towards my right. And as I was sitting on this large rock, I looked down and saw a small treasure chest.

"Open it," I heard a deep voice say.

I opened the treasure chest slowly, and to my surprise I saw gold coins, jewels, crystals, and money – a lot of money inside of this treasure chest!

"Claim it, it's yours," the deep voice said.

And so, I did.

I claimed it then saw the word 'wealth' float up from the treasure chest and up towards the sky. I saw every single letter clearly:

W-E-A-L-T-H.

"Look closely," the voice said. And I saw the letters rearrange themselves into:

H-E-A-L.

The word 'heal' is embedded in the word 'wealth'.

"You can't create wealth until you heal," I heard the deep voice say.

And then the letters rearranged themselves again to spell:
H-E-A-L T-H-E W-E.

'Heal the We' are the same letters as 'wealth'.

Healing yourself, the I, the I AM, heals the WE (generations, ancestors, and the collective) which creates wealth.

Healing the We creates wealth, and it begins by you choosing to heal your Self.

When I witnessed the unfolding of this profound message, I felt a rush of energy filled with purpose, and I immediately had an inner knowing this is what I'm meant to experience and share with the world.

Healing the WE creates wealth, generational wealth, and it begins with *you* believing it's possible. Healing your inner world and loving every phase of the journey creates a better outer world, the New Earth.

And the world needs more love and healing, wouldn't you agree?

'Prayer for the World' written by Howard Wills

God, for me, my family, our entire lineage, and all humanity throughout all time, past, present, and future please help us all forgive each other, forgive ourselves, forgive all people and all people forgive us completely and totally, now and forever please God, thank you God, Amen.

Fill us all with your love and give us all complete peace now and forever please God, thank you God, Amen.

Help us all love each other and love ourselves, be at peace with each other and be at peace with ourselves now and forever please God, thank you God, Amen.

God, we give you our love and thank you for your constant love and blessings. We appreciate and respect all your creations and we fill all your creations with our love.

We thank you God for your love.
We thank you God for our lives.
We thank you God for all life.

We thank you God for all your creations.

We love you God, thank you for loving us.
We love you God, thank you for loving us.
We love you God, thank you for loving us.
Thank you God, Amen.

God, please open, bless, empower, expand, lead, guide, direct, and protect me, my family, and all humanity throughout all time past, present, and future now and forever please God, thank you God, Amen.

Thank you God, Amen.

Chapter 7
Unlock the Alchemist
Within You

There's power in knowing who you are because you unlock the alchemist within you.

You awaken and your light reignites and shines for you to see yourself and for you to be seen in your greatness and Divinity.

The process of being known is a journey of alchemy.

And to be honest, I didn't know what alchemy really meant, even after reading *The Alchemist* by Paul Coelho, I still couldn't really connect to what the experience was all about. It wasn't until I experienced alchemy wholeheartedly from the inside that I understood we are all alchemist, with the power to transform and co-create our realities.

While writing this book, the word 'alchemy' was coming up repeatedly for me. At one point I paused to ask, what does alchemy mean to me? So, I dissected the word al-chem-y and realised the word 'chemical' is embedded in the middle.

Alchemy is an inner chemical reaction, transforming energies from lower vibrational emotions to elevated, higher vibrational emotions. Energy cannot be destroyed, only shifted, and transformed. And since emotions are energies in motion, you can alchemize fear into love, shame into forgiveness, anger into acceptance, guilt into compassion, and pain into freedom.

You are an alchemist, and that power awakens when you choose to know your Self, and when you dive into knowing yourself, you can face the fears, darkness; and with grace and courage, alchemize it all into love and light. From mud to lotus flower, you are an alchemist alchemizing to heal and shine brighter.

Inner Alchemy is a daily practice of returning to love and remembering who you are.

When you return to love, you get to serve humanity with love. That's the main purpose of living this life – return to love, the true essence of who you are, and serve the world. At the end of the day, that's what co-creating is all about. It's not about the amount of money in your bank account, it's not about your title or credentials, it's not about anything materialistic. To live is to receive yourself, as you are in totality, wholeheartedly.

Return to love and serve. Serve Mother Earth. Serve each other. Serve the We. Heal and return to love within yourself to heal and serve the We. And if every person chose to know themselves on a deeper level, chose to be stewards of their own hearts, to heal and love every cell, plus forgive, and share the joy of gratitude, then I believe the world will brighten with everyone's light shining.

That's the journey of alchemy.

Fear-based behavioural patterns led me here – it was all a catalyst for me to dive deeper into my Self and gain clarity that it was all an illusion – an illusion playing a role to forget who I really am.

So, without the fear-based behavioural patterns to fill a void deep inside of me means I'm not identified by anything. I'm not a healer. I'm not physical therapist. I'm not any titles.

I simply AM – infinite, cosmic, multidimensional, led by my heart's wisdom.

I am present in every now moment. That's who I choose to be.

Present in my power. Present in my Divinity. Present vibrating at higher frequencies.

Present.

Simply being.

Breathing in and out.

Co-existing with everything around me.

Present.
Being.
Breathing.
Living.

Connecting to the truth of who I AM...

A breath of life – exploring, navigating, alchemizing, ascending, evolving, aligning, grounding, surrendering, rebirthing, shining light, and breathing in life.

And connecting to the power of breathing while you're healing and returning to love is a form of alchemy too.

You inhale oxygen, exhale carbon dioxide and your nervous system shifts from sympathetic-driven (fight-or-flight) to parasympathetic (rest-digest-rejuvenate) when you focus on longer exhalation, a state in which the body and mind slow down, allowing you to feel more at ease, receptive, calm, and present.

Moving your body with the intention to release and let go of what no longer serves you while at the same time believing your body is strong and healthy unlocks the alchemist within you. Conscious eating and connecting to what you're putting in and on your body is alchemy too.

Recreating new beliefs so you can receive what you believe is an inner chemical reaction because you shift from feeling confined to feeling expanded by choosing to experience a better reality. It's an energetic shift you get to experience daily.

Choosing and deciding what's best for your soul's evolution is alchemy. You become aware of Self – mind, body, heart, and spirit – which means you're awake, awake to see your Self through the lens of love.

And when you're aware and awake to see yourself, you get to receive yourself. You receive. Your heart opens to receive, and you receive the magic of your heart.

You receive Mother Earth. You receive the sun, moon, and stars. You receive the wind, water, and heat from the passion brewing inside of you to live your life authentically in full expression.

You receive yourself. And by receiving yourself fully, you receive another – another person's love and light, wisdom, medicine, support, and encouragement to continue moving forward on your journey of alchemy.

And then you get to integrate it all.

Feel the elevated emotions and expansive beliefs spreading throughout your entire body. Imagine your life unfolding divinely because you're an energetic match for your heart's desires and more.

Integrate to install the wisdom codes that you gained from your inward journey. Receive the gifts and lessons from alchemizing fear into love, darkness into light.

Live it. Experience it. *Be* it.

Align to your truth daily and become one with your body.

And create. Create beauty. Create a sustainable way of living. Create space for you to reclaim all of you and integrate the light and power of being known fully.

Chapter 8
Embody the Truth
of Who You Are

Em-bodi-ment – a divine alignment with all that is, centred throughout all time and space, radiating an omnipresent energy as a magnetic sovereign being. Embodiment is understanding yourself deeply – present with the essence of your presence, co-creating reality. Embodiment strengthens the journey of self-discovery.

Embody elevated beliefs and perceptions about your Self, your life, and others. Embody the new way of being within your heart and body.

And you become the truth of who you are by embodying the power of your heart. Heart Embodiment is a daily self-love practice amplifying the heart's (and Earth's) electromagnetic power. Your senses heighten, feeling from up above, down below, and all around you with more awareness. Spiritual gifts are activated to support your growth and expansion. And you no longer doubt the intuition of your heart. The mind clears, the body softens and relaxes, trusting you have everything you need within. In flow, magnetizing energetic experiences. Devoting yourself to the practice of self-love transforms your life.

On the morning of November 18, 2021, while staying at a cabin in Mt. Shasta, I tuned into myself because I felt tension in my heart and body, and realised I had a fear of being loved. I feared love.

I felt afraid of love and allowing myself to be loved.

Why?

Because love cracks you wide open. Love is freedom. Love is powerful. Love expands you. And I carried this fear of love in my heart and body for many years and lifetimes. I didn't trust love. I blamed love for betraying me. I shamed love for abandoning me. And I hid from love with a thick heart wall believing I was too much and difficult to love. But love has a way of sneaking in. Love encapsulated my heart in the space of stillness and reminded me I am love and created to love and be loved. I am the embodiment of love. And receiving myself by connecting to my heart is the greatest act of self-love. The truth is love doesn't betray or abandon. Fear does. Fear pulls you away from self-love and empowerment.

I felt the fear of love fully and became aware that this fear related to all of my left-sided pain and heartache; related to why I felt uncomfortable receiving gifts, support, money, and love from others; explains why I built walls and self-sabotaged and attracted lies, deception, and infidelity; and it's also why I cheated on my heart so many times.

I feared love and fearing love meant I feared myself – afraid of my own power; scared of expansion and being stretched beyond my comfort zone, and glitched with experiencing a lot of money and abundance. So, to be able to dive in and feel into this fear, I got to shift it, transform it, and alchemize it into being open to love – allowing myself to be love and receive love from deep within to nourish my heart.

Feeling this freedom and leaning into this new belief and story activated my cells and it spread throughout my entire body. It felt like electricity flowing through me as I surrendered into receiving love and being loved –being loved by my family, colleagues and friends; being loved by Mother Earth and all her elements; being loved by the Universe, stars, and planets; being loved by money, joy, and abundance; being loved by wealth and vitality; being loved by *all* – because I AM love. Love is the essence of who I AM.

And now I get to embody the truth wholeheartedly, embody love and being loved in every single cell of my heart and body.

This is embodiment – allowing every single cell to absorb love, absorb joy and happiness, absorb wealth and prosperity because you believe you're worthy and deserving; because you're aware of the power of being known and understand the power goes beyond you – generations before and after you – and it travels to shift the world around you because you chose to embody the truth of who you are – and who you are is worth knowing.

It all comes back full circle. Allowing myself to know myself on a cellular level and be known allows others to know themselves on a deep cellular level to be seen and known. We are all here guiding each other home – home to our hearts, home to our bodies, and home to the truth of who we are.

Special day today!
A really special day.
I woke up this morning with gratitude and realised I get to know myself all over again. I'm shifting, quantum leaping and every morning, I'm a new person.

So, who am I?
I AM LIGHT.
That's who I AM.

So, when we embody the power of the heart, we shine our light for others to see the light within themselves.

Heart Embodiment brightens your light and sparks the world around you – like glitter!

Josh's Journey

What was the catalyst in your life for you to know yourself on a deeper level and share your gifts with the world?

When I think about the catalyst in my life for me to know myself on a deeper level and share my gifts with the world, it seems like a big question. But as big of a question as it is, my response is crystal clear and comes rushing in and I'm able to pinpoint a certain moment.

It started as a normal Thursday. I was a junior in high school getting ready for football practice. I got to the field early to stretch and loosen up because a couple weeks earlier, I sustained a hard hit to my right quad in a game and the deep bone bruise was not getting better. That night at practice, I took a teammate's knee directly to the soft spot and saw the stars. I remember rolling on the field in pain, our team trainer coming over and telling me to suck it up.

But as I was driving home that night, it started swelling up and the pain became severe. I had to drive with my left foot the last couple miles home. I sat on the couch and stayed there until I had my uncle and dad help carry me to my room.

My parents were trying to find some sleeping pills or pain killers to help me try to get some rest and sleep it off, and in hindsight I can be thankful that their search came up short. My entire upper leg swelled and became hard as a rock. The pain became unbearable. Finally, we made the call to go to the ER to get some ice and pain pills to help me get through the night – so we thought.

After the ER doctor quickly diagnosed my condition as compartment syndrome, he got the orthopaedic surgeon on call paged in to prep for surgery. He explained to me and my parents that I had a rare injury that needed an operation right away. Due to the swelling in my quad, my entire muscle compartment filled with blood and was cutting off blood flow from the rest of my leg. It was a matter of hours before the muscles in my entire leg would die off resulting in the need for amputation.

That was a lot for my 17-year-old morphine-filled mind to take in, as I was more concerned at the time about being at the hospital and not being able to study for my biology test the next day. Thankfully there's a simple procedure known as a fasciotomy they could do to alleviate the pressure, stop the bleeding, and restore normal function to my leg. So less than 90 minutes after arriving to the ER, I was wheeled into the operating room.

The surgery was a success. And I woke up with a 10-inch incision mark up the side of my leg with 18 staples holding it together. Something else happened during that surgery that I would come to uncover a few days later.

After being discharged from the hospital, I sat at home in my bed and was able to begin to process what had just happened in the unexpected whirlwind of the previous few

117

days. I felt called to pick up a pen and paper. I grabbed loose graph paper from my backpack and started scribbling words. The words began flowing like an open faucet. I started writing what took the form of a poem. A spoken word poem, designed to be read aloud. I filled the front and back of the paper in one swift move, not stopping the pen flowing for one moment, and not crossing out a single letter.

After writing it, I hobbled to the kitchen on crutches to my mom and said, "Hey mom, I'm not quite sure what I just wrote, but can I read it to you?"

She was in tears after listening to me read the poem. I was a bit shocked too, I honestly didn't know what half of the words I wrote meant at the time, but I knew it was powerful. After sharing with the rest of my family, my parents suggested that I record myself performing the poem so we could share it with other people. We had the idea of recording it in an empty hospital room at the hospital where they did my surgery. After help from a family friend who worked at the hospital, we were put in touch with the right person who helped us set it up.

While my dad filmed me performing the poem, someone who worked at the hospital overheard and was moved to emotion. She had me send the video to her and it was eventually shared with the head of PR for the Scripps Hospital. Next thing I know, I'm being interviewed for the cover patient story of the quarterly hospital magazine and invited to events, galas, and functions to share my story and my poem.

While that was cool to see something like this come from my injury, at the time I was still severely bummed because my recovery meant that I couldn't participate in my team's basketball season that winter. Turns out there was something greater in store and my shovel was about to hit another hidden gem.

My class adviser was someone I had a great relationship with. He happened to be the drama teacher. When he knew I now had time freed up because of no basketball, he took it as an opportunity to invite me to audition for our spring drama production of Shakespeare's "Much Ado About Nothing."

I laughed at the idea of it initially, to his face. The thought of me in a Shakespeare play was almost as ludicrous as the ER doctor telling me that I needed surgery to save the function of my leg that night in November 2011. But he told me that when students auditioning for one of the lead roles, the direction he gave them was to act more 'Josh Church.' He said the role was built for me and he thought that I would really love it.

Because I valued our relationship I auditioned for the part. I ended up getting the role. At the time it was something to fill my time and keep me engaged. It would evolve to certainly be one of the most special things I was a part of throughout my high school career. It invigorated my passion for the arts, reading, and writing. I worked closely with one of our teachers who was our dramaturge, helping break down the words of Shakespeare so we could bring them to life. It stimulated my intellectual curiosity in a way that was new to me.

I shined on stage under the lights and felt at home, like a fish swimming in water. Being part of a team in a way that was similar to sports but different was such a spectacular feeling. I started to suspect that this compartment syndrome thing may have been a course corrective catalyst for me to uncover certain gifts within myself and set me on a mission to share them with the world.

And then that summer, the culminating event took place to confirm my suspicions.

Scripps Hospital flew me out to deliver the keynote patient story to their system wide doctor conference. I stood up on stage in a large hotel ballroom, in front of a room of 1,000 doctors from all over the country and shared my story and my poem. My mom was there with me, and she was asking me before if I was nervous, but I remember for some odd reason being completely not nervous. It was my story, my words, I knew it all and it felt so aligned.

I got up on stage and something just took over me – I was present, comfortable, confident, and totally in my zone. And it felt so right. My words resonated deeply as I received a standing ovation from the entire room. It was then I understood the power of words and stories and how they can move emotions on a soul level. It was one of those light bulb moments where it felt like the runway was lighting up for me to continue to show up to serve others in this way.

The breadcrumbs of my injury led me to be able to finally look at my compartment syndrome as a blessing. Rather than despise the crappy injury, I could feel a sense of gratitude for all that it had led me to. And in that moment, true healing occurred.

It wasn't the first or the last of my physical injuries and challenges. I've experienced and overcome a whole lot in my short few decades exploring being human on planet earth. It began within the first few minutes after I was born, when my lung collapsed. It continued through my boyhood when I got to know "Chuck," the guy at the orthopaedic office who puts casts on, on a first name basis. It continued through ACL reconstruction surgery, compartment syndrome, and a botched appendectomy that resulted in internal bleeding and required multiple blood transfusions.

Thankfully as I sit here today, I am not only healthy, but I am experiencing a level of health, vitality, and well-being that I didn't think was possible. In fact, it was ONLY possible through each and every apparent roadblock that I can now see was a speed ramp. The setback was the opening act for the comeback.

Each health challenge provided the catalyst for deeper growth at that stage. Physically, mentally, spiritually, emotionally. It matured me. Pulled me inward to get to know myself in an intimate way. Gave me opportunities to define myself. Forged a level of inner strength, grit, leadership and determination that I couldn't have gotten any other way. It quite literally forced me on a journey of health and wellness that led me to places, people, and experiences around the world that I could only have dreamt of including becoming a certified Yoga Instructor and Wim Hof Breathwork instructor. It fuelled motivation to summit mountains, run marathons, and train for Ironman triathlons. It allowed me to discover gifts of writing, speaking, performing, and creativity that lied dormant, revealing a sense of purpose to share that with others. It launched me on a career path of helping others on their growth journey sharing my perspectives, insights, and takeaways from my own experiences. It led me to launch my newest business, where we are on a mission to help people get the edge on their recovery, on their performance, on winning the day. Developing products, software, and services that help people deepen their relationship with themselves. To stress less, achieve more, and feel more alive. To develop a healthier body and stronger mind.

Being fuelled on this path is invigorating. Its alignment and clarity to the highest degree. And I know that whatever challenges, curveballs, or plot-twists life throws at me, I'll be ready to step back in the batter's box and take another swing. Rather than allowing adversity to define me, I will continue to use it as an opportunity to define myself – trusting that each moment can be a catalyst that take me deeper within myself, polish up buried gifts, and share it with the world.

Invitation

Write down a fear that's been on repeat. One that continues to show up in your life and has confined you into going bigger and expanding. And notice where you feel it in your body as you're connecting and diving into this fear. What are you most afraid of? And breathe into the area of your body where it feels uncomfortable and restrictive. Notice how you feel and allow the emotions to flow through you.

Then ask, "Is this my truth? Is this fear and what I'm afraid of my truth? And do I wish to continue living out this fear that's been trapped in my body?"

Be honest with yourself without judgement.

If you wish to free yourself from this fear, then what is your new story? What do you choose to believe in so you can receive it in your body? Write it out. Say it out loud. Declare your new story. Notice how you feel. Is the tension in your body dissolving? Breathe into yourself and exhale the fear. Breathe it out and allow it to leave your body and intend Mother Gaia to absorb it so she can repurpose it to grow trees, plants, and beauty around you. Breathe in your new story and breathe out the fear and worry.

Continue this practice of breathing in and exhaling until you feel every single cell absorb your new elevated belief and story. Feel the lightness and sense of freedom you are now co-creating within your heart.

Allow this heightened feeling to spread throughout your entire body. Bathe yourself in it. Marinate in it – the *it* being your true essence. The *it* being the freedom you're co-creating for yourself and generations before and after you. The *it* being the love you're pouring into yourself now.

Embody it.

Receive it.

Embody it daily with thoughts, words, and intentional actions that continue to ignite this feeling of lightness you're experiencing right now in this moment.

Breathe it in! Breathe it *all* in and believe you're worthy of experiencing this.

And now you have this heart embodiment, self-love practice to return to anytime you feel pain, a glitch in your nervous system, any time you feel 'off'. Return to yourself, dive in, explore, feel every emotion and exhale. Then breathe in your new belief and story and embody – embody the elevated feeling in every single cell of your heart and body and become it in every single now moment.

The Universe is orchestrating in my favour for the greater good. So, yes, I surrender. I let go of the reins. I release the need to control. And trust. Trust I have everything I need. Trust I'm right where I need to be. Trust it's all unfolding in divine timing. Trust it's all happening for me. Trust.

And I'd rather trust than resist. Resistance creates tension. Creates pain. Creates suffering. Resisting is not in alignment with the magic of the present moment. Resistance delays receiving the magic and abundance that surrounds me daily.

So, I open my heart and choose to trust daily – trust in every now moment.

Trust with an open heart, ready for it all – ready to receive what the Universe is orchestrating for me and for all. Receive with an open heart. And believe in the magic of it all!

Life and Death Embodiment

Death.

It's part of knowing yourself.

Death is part of living. And death co-exists in harmony with life so that you can *live* fully.

I connected to the essence of Death on November 4, 2021. I received news that morning that a dear friend of mine passed, transitioned to the Heavens from a car accident. He was like a soul brother to me. And I was in shock he transitioned so quickly. I knelt down on the floor crying, wondering what to do. Do I fly back to Texas to be with my family and stop my California journey, or do I continue moving forward with what I'm guided to do here? As I was feeling every fear and emotion, I heard his voice tell me, "Keep going. Keep going with your mission." And in that moment, I felt a knowing he'll be supporting me with moving forward. At the time, I was staying at a dear family friend's house in Santa Ynez and I shared the news with her. She offered to go on a walk, and I knew I had to play sound with my Alchemy Crystal Bowl. So, later that day, we walked onto an open field and found spot for us to sit, breathe, feel, connect, and release.

I brought my Alchemy Crystal Sound bowl made of Abalone (the sound bowl is Note D sharp which connects to the sacral chakra). I closed my eyes, entered a deep meditative state, and felt surprised with what I received.

I saw Death as a Goddess, swaying her body from side to side. She felt pure and divine dressed in black and violet and she said:

"Thank you for honouring me for I am part of living. I coexist with life. I'm not a destroyer or something to be afraid of. I'm an alchemist, a transformer, and I'm here to remind you to live your life fully. I am beauty in raw form. Yes, I'm blamed, shamed, and judged, and perceived as taking life away. The truth is, I add to life, creating space for more light to enter this place. I am not fear. I co-exist with life. And I'm here as a reminder to live your life. Mother Earth embodies life and death within Her. Death and rebirth are a constant. You, too, embody life and death within you. Your cells die and regenerate for you to live this life. Set me free so I can fulfil my divine purpose. No need to be afraid of me. I co-exist with life as part of living. Honour me and set me free in my Divinity and live your life fully."

This message came through me as I harmonised with sound resonating from the crystal sound bowl. I felt tears stream down my face as I felt Death in her beauty and essence. Peace spread throughout my entire being, gaining awareness and understanding Death's purpose. She is part of life and is here to remind us to live our lives fully.

After the experience felt complete, I opened my eyes and sat in silence for a while, allowing everything to marinate. My dear friend was sitting in front of me holding space. She then saw a deer, a female deer, walk out into the field in front of us. The deer stopped and looked at us for a while. I could feel the deer's presence and energy, and, in that moment, I felt everything *is* alive. Everything around me is alive and I felt in in every single cell of my body.

The sun was shining on my face, the oak trees surrounding us, the birds flying up above, the wind blowing through us, the grass, the soil, the deer looking right at us – everything felt alive. Everything *is* alive because death co-exists *with* life.

Connecting to the essence of Death that day was an experience I'll forever remember. Rather than feeling like a part of me was lost (like I did when my cousin died), I gained peace understanding the purpose of it all – the role death plays in our lives and how I get to perceive Her. And I choose to perceive death as part of life, alchemizing, transforming, and beautiful. I'm no longer afraid of death, no longer attached to the fear of losing someone. I set death free (and myself) to fulfil Her divine purpose as part of living.

I perceive every person's presence as a gift. And life gifted us this life. So, whenever one transitions into the Heavens, I no longer view it as a loss because life gifted us their presence and I get to connect with the memories in my heart – at peace and free.

Death also relates to your past self dying. As you get to know yourself, you let go of old programs, limiting beliefs, and stories that once defined you. You begin to shift your identity and release the old to create space for the new. Just like your cells die and regenerate, so does your soul – and you can experience grieving as you let go of the past version of you that you felt comfortable with for so long.

Knowing yourself can feel uncomfortable because you're choosing to face the darkness that's deep within your subconscious. But you're worth being known, even the dark aspects of yourself, because you can shine light and illuminate that space where darkness hides within you. And when darkness lightens, you shed that old part of you and release all attachments as you ascend and spiral upwards vibrating at the frequency of love and enlightenment.

So, allow the grieving process to happen. Feel it and don't rush yourself out of it. Write a letter to your younger self that was holding onto fear and limiting beliefs so tightly. Let him/her go with peace, love, forgiveness, and gratitude. Your past self served a purpose and now it's time to let him/her go the deeper you go into knowing your soul.

Set yourself free from the past. And let loved ones go who have passed. Forgive yourself. Pour love into you. And grieve however long you feel the need to. And understand death co-exists in harmony with life so you can live this life fully.

Death and Resurrection

From March–May 2021, I experienced the most intense internal death and resurrection.

In March, I declared out loud, "I'm ready to step into my power!"

"Are you sure?" I heard a voice say in response to my declaration.

And after a pause I responded with a 'YES!'

Little did I know how intense stepping into my power fully was going to go. I've been one step into my power and one step out for so long and to declare I'm ready to step in with both feet meant I needed to face, feel, and heal all the things that no longer resonated with stepping into my power and expansion.

Expansion means a deepening needs to happen – letting go of all the things that have been confining you: self-sabotaging behaviours, childhood and generational traumas, fears, beliefs and perceptions that are not in alignment with divine love, thoughts, lifestyle choices – everything – needed to be felt and alchemized to expand.

Why did I express my readiness out loud??

Because I was done feeling afraid of my own power. I was done fearing the unknown. I was done dimming my own light and playing small. I was done. And I knew I had to be done because my soul's purpose was pulling me to be done. I'm here on a divine mission and I needed to dive deeper and completely surrender to the Divine/God/Source/Universe because their plan is way bigger than ego's. The cosmic plan had already been orchestrating a better, bigger version than I had ever imagined; and for me to fully experience the richness of life, I had to declare that I'm ready and completely surrender – surrender – surrender.

And in the process of surrendering and letting go of attachments and past identities I experienced a rebirth.

I connected to the essence and power of who I AM.

Because when you purge and purify physically, mentally, and emotionally, what's left is the I AM essence. You stop forgetting and remember.

I surrendered and felt the energy of GOD deep inside of me.

I AM GOD.

God is within me.

The energy of God is within me and it's *all* inside of me.

I'm a multi-dimensional cosmic being made of stars and Earth's elements. I am energy, ever-changing and ever-evolving. I am nowhere and everywhere at the same time. I am alive and divinely connected down below, up above, and all around me. I am light. I am the breath of life. I am the heartbeat of the Universe.

I am of the Earth to be in God.

I AM.

And I was reborn – again.

The three-month process felt like I was constantly pulling weeds deep inside of me which all served a purpose as part of my heart-cantered journey so that I can find the precious seed of light representing the I AM deep within my heart.

From 'who am I?' To I am.

From death to resurrection.

So, I can step into my power fully.

Even though the process, which I like to call, 'The Great Purge' felt painful on all levels, it served a grand purpose to be the woman I am becoming.

I gave my power away and it became 'normal' for me. I believed it was the only way to fit in.

And today, I no longer give my power away. I am safe to claim my power, stand in it, embrace it, accept it, and express myself fully without feeling the need to people please and fit in.

I am safe to fully express myself and love myself throughout the entire experience of showing up in my full power and energy – with love.

Everyone is on their own personal journey and I no longer need to dim my light for them to feel comfortable. I can take up space like Mt. Shasta. Take up space and shine – that's magnetic! Mt. Shasta shines her light and people gravitate towards her to experience her high vibe. Mt. Shasta reminds me to be the same – take up space and shine, and people will be magnetized by my presence.

I'm grateful everything (and everyone) is a reflection because it allows me to dive into myself and explore to heal, learn, and receive the gifts of reflection.

I am safe to express myself fully.
I am safe.
I am safe.

And it's more fun that way!

Expressing myself fully feels vibrant, electric, magnetic, attractive, beautiful, powerful, creative, sensual, and intimate.

So, yes, it's worth the experience.

And I didn't experience 'The Great Purge' alone. I asked for support. I connected with a close friend of mine who is a high-level healer and gained the support I needed. Every session together we dove in deep with the intention to alchemize childhood and generational fears and traumas, clear energetic cords and attachments, integrate new beliefs, and awaken the power of love within so I can receive my Self wholeheartedly.

Three intense months of purging and being born again. And I'm grateful I gained support every step of the way.

The journey of knowing yourself is not meant to be experienced alone. It takes a village. The journey is continuous and ever-evolving. And it's worth experiencing because I now get to share the wisdom and medicine from my inner exploration and allow myself to be known fully, known in my rawness and vulnerability.

Because I chose to. I decided. I listened and acted on what was needed. And I allowed myself to be led and guided by my internal compass, trusting I have everything I need within me, and my life continues to unfold with surprises daily.

Trusting and surrendering deeper fuelled me daily, plus, pouring love into me and spreading the energies of light, wisdom, love, wealth, and prosperity is my divine soul mission.

Knowing myself deeply means I'm aware. I'm awake. And writing this book is fulfilling my destiny. I was led and guided to, and I'm grateful you're here to experience a heart-centred journey connecting to Self, Earth, lineage, and love.

Invitation

What part of you needs to die for you to resurrect and live this life fully?

What do you feel and believe you are designed and destined to be?

Create a sacred space for yourself to dive in and explore. Allow the answers to the questions to come up to the surface for you to feel, gain awareness, and discover the truth. Grab a pen and paper and write it out. Let your heart tell you. Lean in. Let go. Surrender. Exhale. And resurrect from the ashes.

Flow and ease.
Exhale and release.
Surrender and simply be.
And flow like the waves of the sea.
In and out. In and out. In and out.
With love and beauty.
And you will see the light within.
The light of your cosmic being, infinite and never-ending.
So, lean back, relax, and receive.
Flow and ease.
Exhale and release.
Surrender and simply be.

Chapter 9
And the Journey Continues

So here we are. At the end of the book journey and at the beginning of your journey of alchemy, diving into yourself to explore the darkness and shine light on the true essence of who you are.

You are love. And there's power in knowing that you are love because you wake up and see your Self through the lens of love without running away anymore. You heal and receive yourself in totality. And strengthen the power of your heart so you can radiate love, light, joy, vitality, and happiness.

Healing and loving your inner world co-creates a healing and loving outer world.

To Heal the We, one must Heal the I, the eye in which you see yourself. Your perception on how you view your Self influences your life's experiences.

The lens in which you see yourself can be blurred by fear, trauma, worry, self-doubt and heartache, shame, guilt, judgement, anger, and frustration.

The lens in which you see yourself can be cleared by love, compassion, courage, connection, trust, and forgiveness, happiness, joy, gratitude, and excitement.

To Heal the I, you must *see* your Self in totality, wholeheartedly, and acknowledge the feelings, emotions, and any discomfort that comes up to the surface so you can connect and nurture what is needed for your soul's evolution.

It all begins with you and you have everything you need to begin anew.

Heartache opened my heart to receive life here and now.

Receive the wisdom of my family lineage.

Receive guidance from God/Great Spirit/ Source/ Universe.

Receive abundance and expansive experiences.

Receive Mother Earth's medicine.

Receive all of me so I can receive you.

Because I am you and you are me – mirrors reflecting the light within.

You are one cell. One cell of many. Together, co-creates your entire being. You are a human being of light, sound, and energy. You are Of the Earth to Be in God so you can see the all-encompassing I AM inside your heart.

You are connected to ALL. So, dive in.

Explore.

Navigate your heart and soul.

And love every phase you're in because there's gold in everything.

You're worth knowing.

Believe me, it's quite a journey meeting yourself on a deeper level daily.

I invite you to deepen within to expand without. Take up space. Receive what you believe and perceive. And allow yourself to experience the richness of life from the inside-out.

The power of being known allows you to connect with the beat of your heart, the sound of your voice, the pause between each breath, the stillness of every moment, and feel the energy of divine love circulating in your blood and spreading throughout every cell of your entire body.

The power of being known is the power of love and the power of love is the power of being known.

Be still, feel, ask, listen, breathe, receive, and know.

And keep going.

Keep going with what's inside of you.

And allow yourself to be known.

Allow yourself to be seen, loved, supported, and heard in your authenticity and vulnerability – with an open heart – intending to shine your light for others to see their light. Honour and celebrate your existence.

Nothing good comes from closing your heart in fear of getting hurt, abandoned, and judged. From fearing the unknown to being known *now* is the journey of self-love. And self-love is the new foundation you can grow from.

The blindfold has been removed and I can now clearly see I have everything I need!

Love is deep inside of me, nourishing me and supporting me daily. And because of Love, I have it all!

Love is everything, infinite, and eternal, flowing divinely, even in the space of darkness.

Love is here, deep inside of me. Love is everything I need!

The fears are dissolving, clearing space for me to clearly see I have everything I need.

I believe in the power of love, and I receive my Self now.

So, journey inward, meet your true Self and open your heart to receive the wisdom and medicine from deep inside you. Surrender, resurrect, and share your gifts, your journey, and your story of becoming.

Alchemize fear.

Integrate your being-ness.

Embody the power of your heart.

And unite with the sacredness of Self, Earth, Lineage, and Love.

Love looked at me and said,
"You're not a failure in my eyes.
Choose me daily.
Let me in.
And I'll embrace you wholeheartedly.
Trust I'm always here healing your heart from
all your fears.
I'm all around you and deep within.
I see you.
I hear you.
I feel you.
Believe you are worthy to receive me for I am you and
you are me.
Choose me daily and let me in."

And so, I did.
I chose Love.
Let Her in.
And met my true Self deep within.